YOUR VAGINA
Everything You Need to Know!

Odile Bagot
Doctor of Gynecology

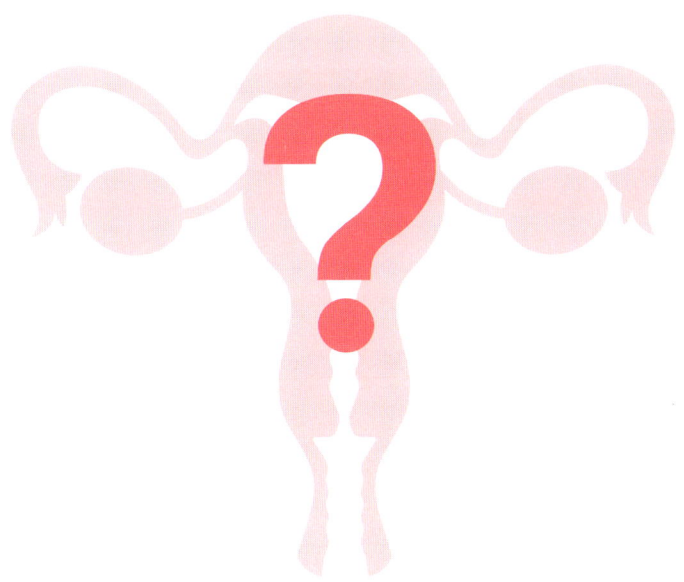

Firefly Books

Contents

Introduction 5

Your Vagina and Its Neighborhood 6

Did You Say Vagina? 6
Where Is It? 6
What Does It Look Like? 10

The Perineum: The Foundation 13

The Vulva: The Temple Entrance 17
The Labia: The Outer Decor 18
The Vestibule: The Foyer 19
The Hymen: The Doorway 20
The Clitoris: The Doorbell 22

The Bladder and Rectum: The Neighbors 24

The Vagina in All Its Forms 26

The Vagina in Everyday Life 26
What Does It Secrete? 26
What Is the Vagina For? 35

The Vagina at All Ages 36
From Birth to Puberty 36
From Puberty to Menopause: Periods 37
Menopause 48

The Vagina and New Life 52
Conception 52
Pregnancy 53
Childbirth 53
Breastfeeding 53

The Vagina for Pleasure! 56
Vaginal Lubrication 56
Vaginal Orgasm 57
What About the G Spot? 60
Sex Toys 63
Vaginal Flatulence 65

The Vagina and Contraceptives 66
    The Pill 67
    Vaginal Rings 68
    Desogestrel Implants and Pills 70
    IUDs 71
    Condoms 75
    Diaphragms and Spermicides 78

Vaginal Problems 82

Vaginismus 82
Pain During Sex 86
    Deep Pain 86
    Superficial Pain 90
Prolapse 95
    How Do You Avoid a "Fall"? 98
    Perineal Rehabilitation 99
    Surgery 100
Cervical Diseases 102
Uterine Diseases 104
Vulvovaginitis 106
    Mycosis (Yeast Infections) 107
    Vaginosis 109
    The "Outsiders" 110
Sexually Transmitted Infections 113
    Chlamydia 114
    Ureaplasma and Mycoplasma Infection 116
    Trichomoniasis 116
    Gonorrhea 117
    Human Papillomavirus Infection 118
    Genital Herpes 120
    Syphilis 121

Conclusion 123
Index 124
Table of Illustrations 125

Introduction

The vagina. You likely barely know this intimate side of yourself, and you'll never be able to see it in its entirety, unless you are both a gynecologist and part-time circus contortionist. You're no doubt curious about it, but you wouldn't dream about asking any questions. Hidden behind that one word — which you may be uncomfortable saying and refer instead to "down there" — lies this largely misunderstood subject of fantasies and beliefs. If you're here, it is because you want to know more about this mysterious organ, whose secrets seem, pardon the expression, impenetrable. So, are you ready to go on a journey to the depths of your intimate self?

Your Vagina and Its Neighborhood

▌Did You Say Vagina?▐

There's no shame in saying those three syllables! Of course, it's not a topic to bring up with perfect strangers during a night out. However, it's important to feel free to learn more about this misunderstood organ, without a sense of taboo or embarrassment.

Let's begin by answering this seemingly simple question: what is the vagina? It is a part of the female anatomy that we speak very little, and often poorly, about — and when we do, we often make mistakes. The vagina is not the vulva nor the uterus nor anything else. It is a semi-open structure that contracts and dilates depending on the circumstances (sexual intercourse, childbirth, etc.) and, together with the vulva, uterus, fallopian tubes and ovaries, forms the female reproductive system, which is largely located inside the body.

The vagina is tucked away, nestled between the bladder and the rectum.

Where Is It?

Do you know exactly where your vagina is? To find it, let's take a closer look at how the female body is made up, from the inside to the lower abdomen (or pelvis, to use the medical term). The vagina is found between the bladder and the rectum — and all three are supported by the pelvic floor (the perineum).

Did You Say Vagina? | 7

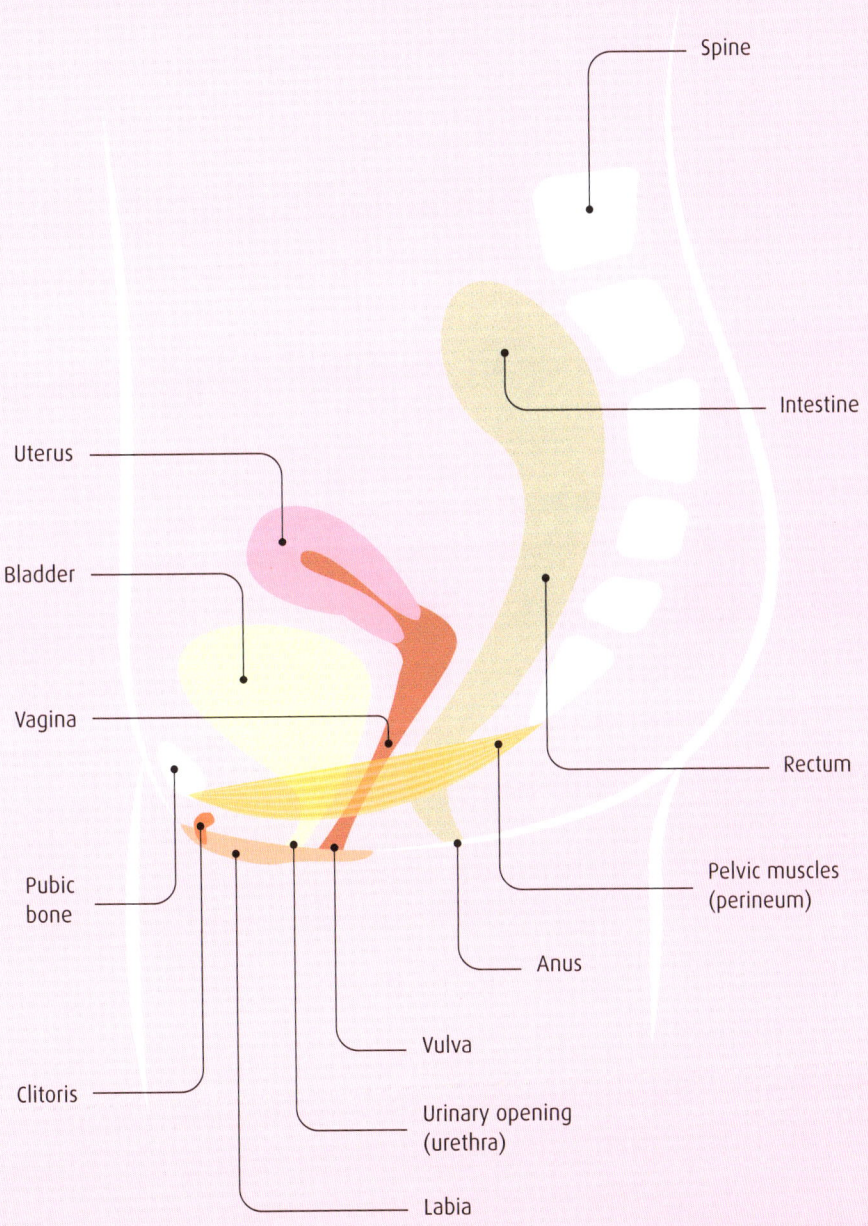

The Female Reproductive System
(sectional view)

The vagina, which measures only about 4 inches (10 cm) long, is found between the vulva and the vaginal fornix, where the cervix comes to a point. Hence, the vagina and the uterus don't "communicate" directly with each other because they are separated by a "security gate"! In fact, the cervix is securely closed, and the uterus and ovaries are not in the same space as the vagina, but are instead in the abdominal cavity. The uterus is linked to the sacrum (the bottom of the spine) by uterosacral ligaments, which help to keep the vagina suspended above the perineum and stop it from bunching up.

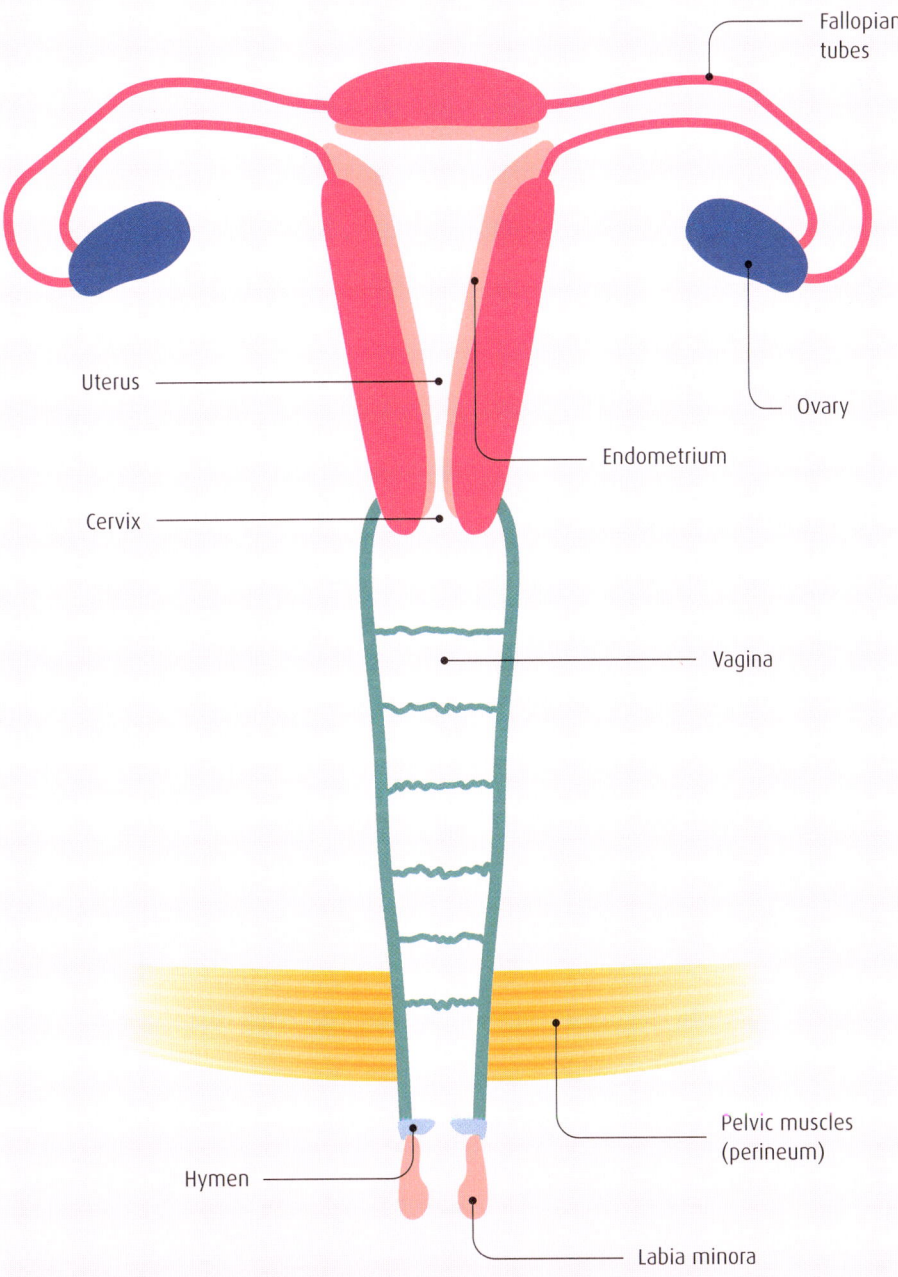

What Does It Look Like?

You may have heard that the vagina is like a cave. **Wrong!** The vagina is not a cavity. In fact, its walls touch when at rest. However, it is the elasticity of its walls that allows a baby, a penis, a tampon or a finger to pass through. The vagina is neither big nor small; it adapts and opens when necessary. The vagina is separated from the vulva by the hymen, a membrane with a perforated center, that sits about ½ inch (1 cm) inside the opening of the vagina. You may have also heard that the hymen completely closes off the vagina before having sex for the first time. **Wrong again!** The hymen is not an armored door; it is flexible and can let in a finger or a tampon without tearing.

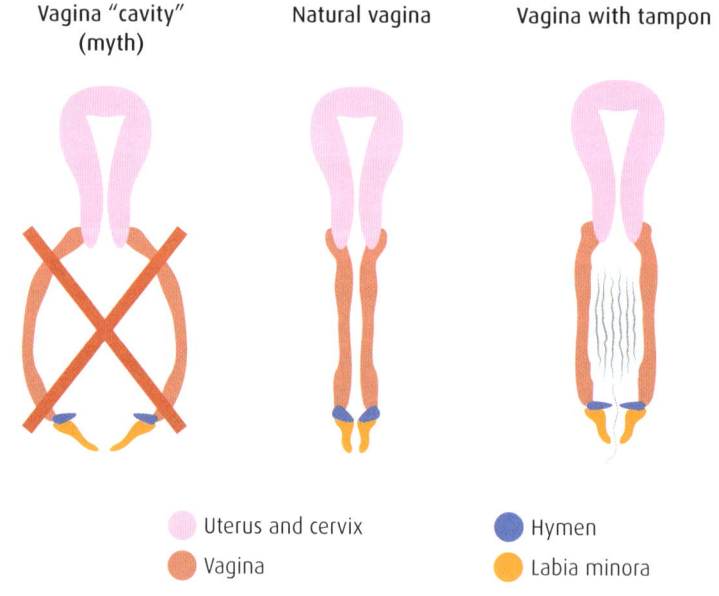

The Vagina and Perineum

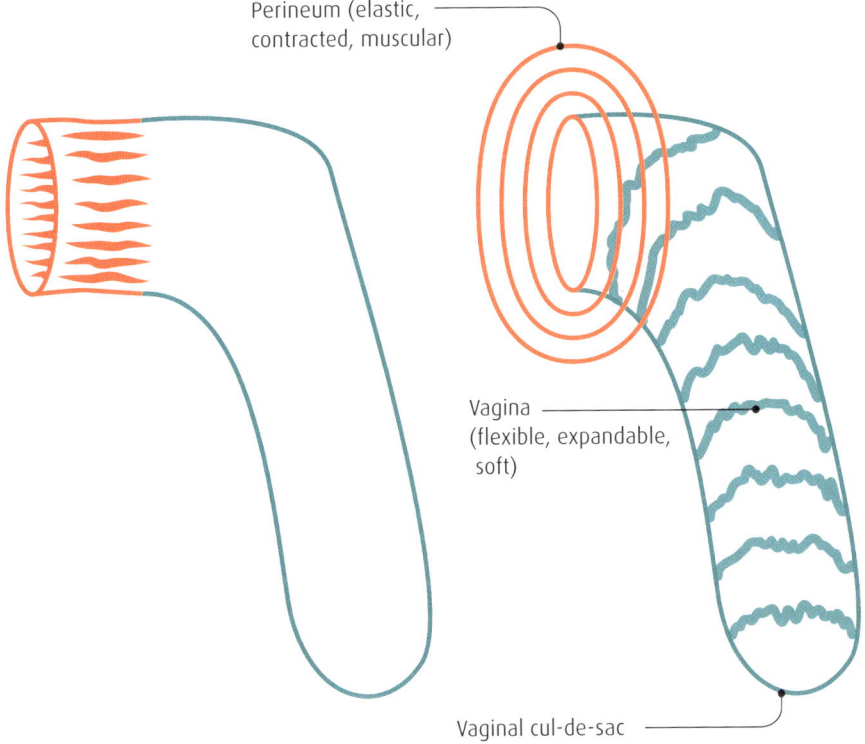

The consistency and shape of the vagina somewhat resemble that of a sock. Yes, you read that correctly! The narrowed and relatively contracted top section (in orange in the above image) is the perineum. Slightly tilted, it extends downward toward the vagina (the main section in blue) and ends at the tip of the vaginal cul-de-sac, where it connects to the cervix. Lastly, from end to end, the vagina lies flat against itself.

The first inch or so of the vagina's walls are a little rough and irregular, and they become smoother farther up the vagina. When menopause begins, those "wrinkles" smooth out. When you squeeze your vagina, you may notice only the opening contracts — that's the perineum muscles working — because the vagina itself lacks muscles.

Mucus, by definition, is always wet, but this wetness varies based on a woman's age, vaginal flora and hormone levels; during pregnancy, for example, women have higher levels of estrogen and an increase in vaginal fluids. Inversely, during menopause, a lack of hormones is responsible for the vagina's relative dryness.

The Perineum: The Foundation

The what? The perineum is a relatively unknown muscle in the human body. Contrary to what you might think, it's not just for women.

This muscle structure, located between the anus and the outer genitals, and the pelvic bone in greater depth, is also present in males. The perineum is like a hammock, stretched between the pubic and coccyx bones. It supports everything in the pelvis (the bladder, uterus, vagina and rectum) and, in the abdominal cavity, the intestines. For a better understanding, imagine the bottom of a big bag with three holes, one for the urethra to expel urine, one for the rectum for stools and one for the vagina. The etymology of "perineum" comes from "to evacuate by orifice." Not very glamorous, but particularly practical. The perineum plays a fundamental role in bladder and bowel continence, as well as sex, regulating the closure of the urethra, anus and vagina.

> **The perineum, or pelvic floor, supports the bladder, uterus and rectum.**

14 | The Perineum: The Foundation

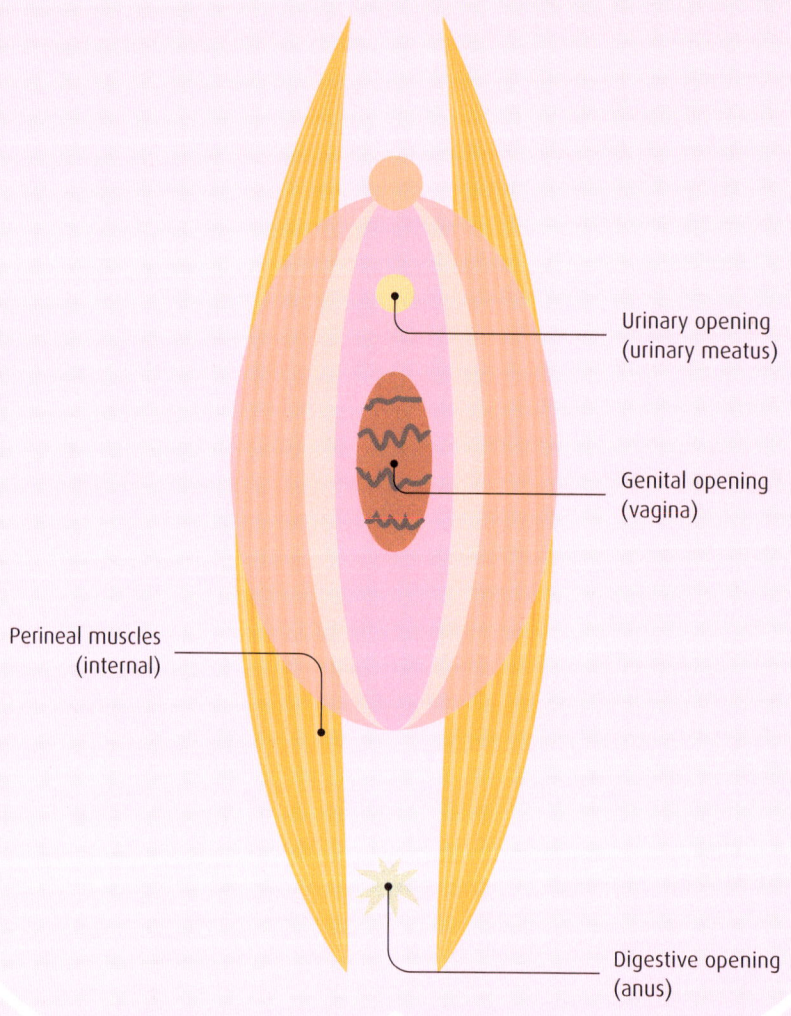

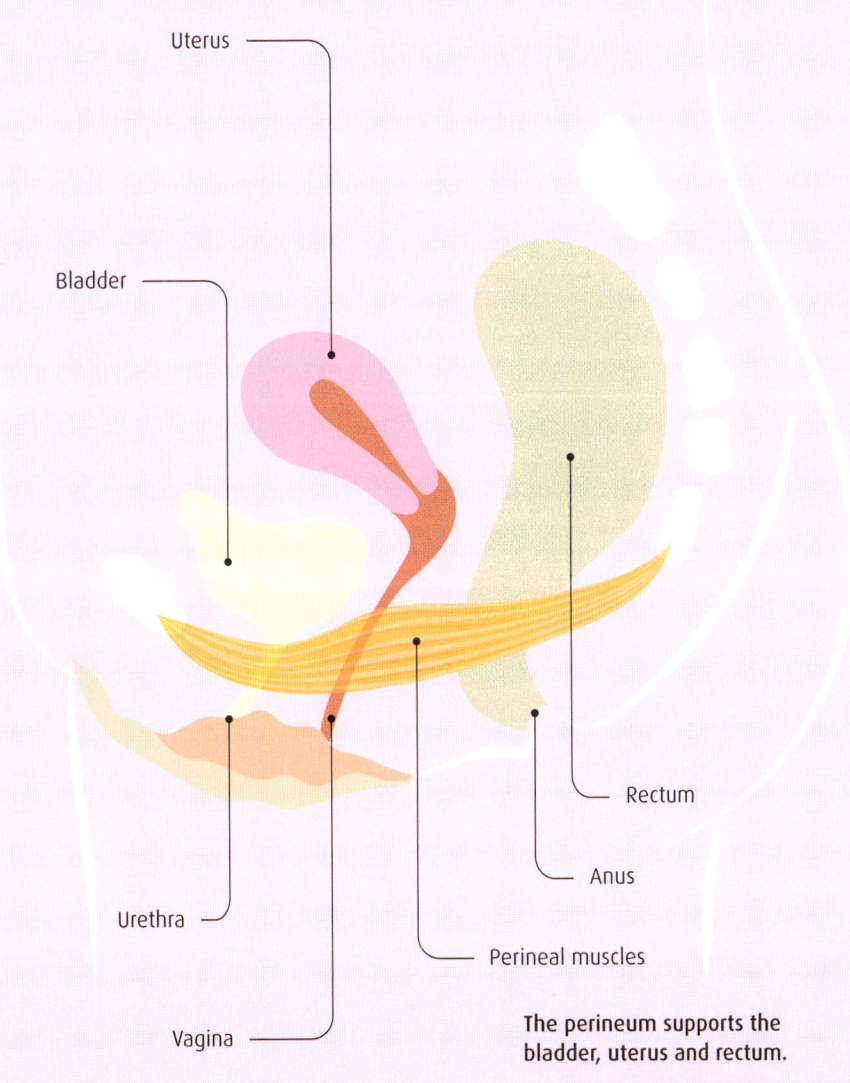

Since the perineal muscles are deep inside the pelvis, it's impossible to see or touch them. However, it is quite possible to feel and engage them, like when you hold the urge to go to the bathroom, for example.

The perineum acts as the bladder's emergency sphincter.

The pelvic floor (another name for the perineum) is essential for both the posture of the pelvis and the support of internal organs. It fully compensates for the absence of vaginal muscles and helps the vagina contract. The bladder's sphincter acts automatically, without the need to control it. In case of urinary urgency or sphincter failure, the perineum acts as a backup sphincter! If the pelvic floor is in good shape, it also reduces the risk of organ prolapse (after childbirth or during menopause).

You no doubt now understand why it is important to maintain the perineum — to strengthen it, to engage it and to (re)train it. If the perineum is relaxed while you're taking a bath, water can enter the vagina, which you will likely notice as you put on your pants and they become wet. To release the water, squat down, relax your perineum, press your thumb toward the back of your vagina, and then squeeze your perineum while you slowly remove your thumb. Having tonic perineal muscles can be of great value in terms of heightened sensations during sex. Another reason to turn this little-known structure into an Olympic champion!

The Vulva: The Temple Entrance

The vulva is the external part of the female reproductive system. It is composed of the labia minora, labia majora, vestibule, hymen and clitoris.

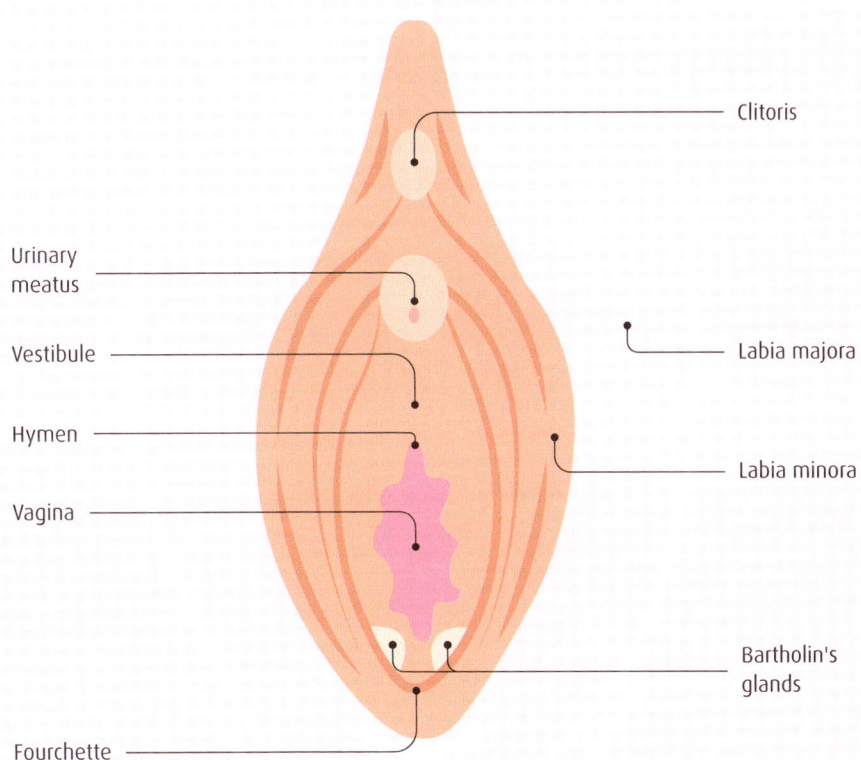

The Vulva
(bottom view)

The Labia: The Outer Decor

The two fleshy, hair-covered labia majora form the outer shape of the vulva, i.e. the visible part of the vulva. In most cases, they completely cover the labia minora. The latter has skin on the outer side, toward the labia majora, and mucus — hence, it's wet — on the inner side, toward the vestibule. This is the hidden part of the vulva.

Labia minora come in all sorts of shapes and sizes. Some women consider surgery to reduce their size. Nymphoplasty (labia minora are also referred to as nympha) is sometimes necessary for those who suffer from hypertrophy of the labia minora, which can interfere with penetration or certain sports (notably cycling and horseback riding). When it comes to cosmetic surgery of normal-sized labia minora — that's a personal choice! However, it's still a surgical procedure so there are always risks. On a side note, however, I can't help wondering why a grown woman would want to change her vulva to look like that of a young girl's. With age, the look of the vulva changes, becoming less dense, less firm and darker.

Nymphoplasty is an operation to reduce the size of the labia minora.

The Vestibule: The Foyer

Ah, the vestibule. So poetic. I love how visual this term is. In a house, the vestibule, or foyer, is the small, beautifully decorated room where you welcome guests, converse with them and exchange compliments before they enter.

A woman's personal vestibule is where some foreplay takes place. This very sensitive area is located precisely between the mucus-facing side of the labia minora and the vaginal opening. Get a mirror, place it on the floor and squat down. Spread your labia minora and you will see the vestibule. Further up, beyond the thin lace of your hymen, you will find your vagina, whose depths are unseen.

The vestibule houses the Bartholin's glands, which help lubricate the vagina during sex. Those glands also have the unfortunate tendency to get blocked, which causes cysts or abscesses to form — an infection is called bartholinitis. If this happens to you, you should consult a doctor.

In case of a vulvovaginal dryness or infection, the pain is stemming from the vestibule, not the vagina itself. On the other hand, the vagina's sensitivity is on another level; it's deeper and harder to feel. Contrary to what you might think, and opposite to the vestibule, the vagina is not very sensitive.

The Hymen: The Doorway

The "intact" hymen (that is, before any penetrative sex) is a thin membrane, measuring $1/32$ to $1/16$ inch (1–2 mm) thick (about the thickness of a quarter) and perforated in the center. It's kind of like a soft ring attached to the vagina wall, separating the vagina from the vestibule. However, you can insert a finger, and the hymen will delicately encase it. When having sex for the first time, the hymen usually tears radially about $1/16$ to $1/8$ inch (2–3 mm), all around the ring. It then forms a thin membrane that hides the vagina from view. Contrary to popular belief, it doesn't always tear during the first sexual encounter; sometimes it just becomes stretched out and doesn't produce the anticipated bleeding, even if the young woman was a virgin.

The Hymen Before and After the First Sexual Encounter

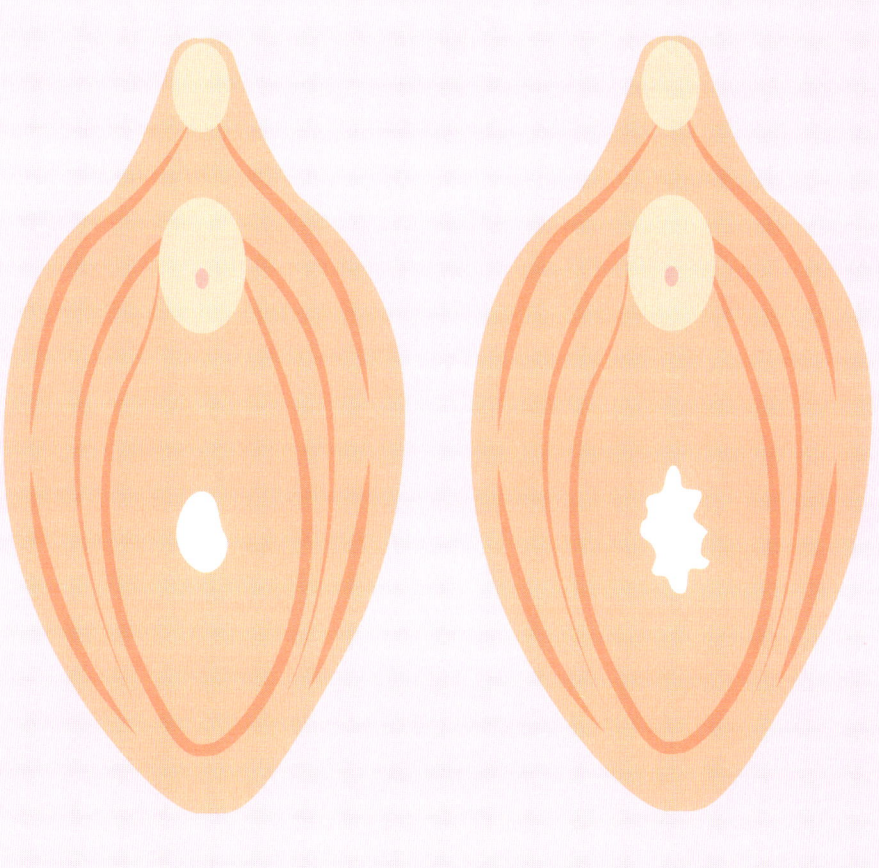

Before   After

The Clitoris: The Doorbell

In ancient Greek, the term clitoris means "small hill." Not far off, right? Most women have located this small, firm button, found just above the urinary meatus and close to the pubic bone. However, few know that it is much bigger than what they see and extends toward the labia majora. Also, the part you can touch, the clitoris gland, is only the tip of the iceberg; the rest of the clitoris lies along the vestibule.

The clitoris is extremely sensitive, a grand master of arousal and the provider of most female orgasms, either alone or in tandem with the vagina. During sex, it swells and erects, but contrary to its male counterpart, the penis, it does not ejaculate — that's the job of the Skene glands, found along the urethra.

The Clitoris
(internal view)

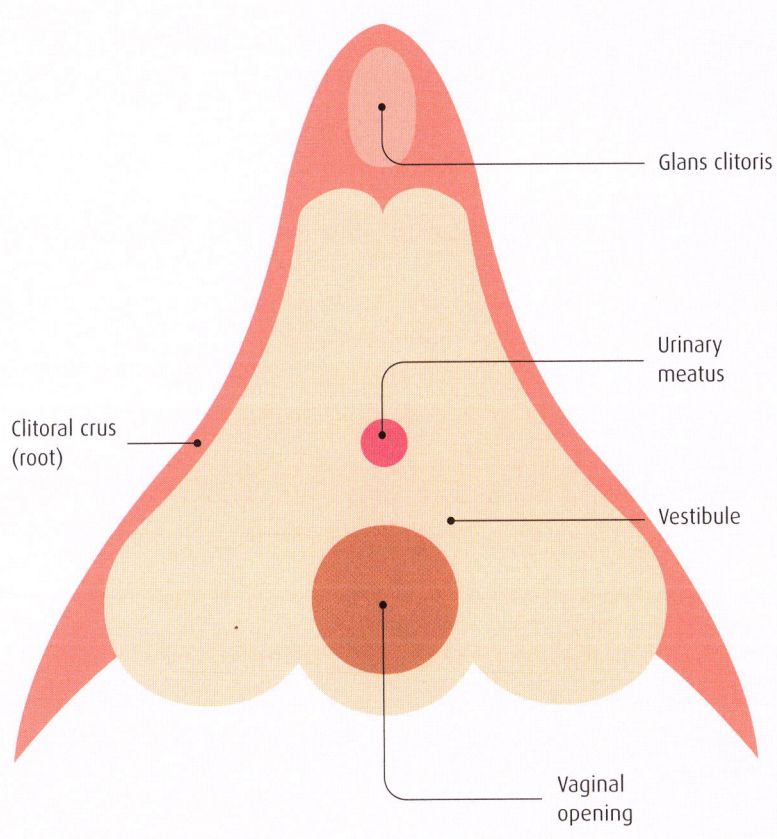

The Bladder and Rectum: The Neighbors

The bladder and the rectum are both closely connected to the vagina.

The bladder, uterus, fallopian tubes, ovaries and rectum are pelvic organs. While the vagina is open toward the outside of the body, it also plays a part in the structure of the pelvis. The bladder wall toward the front and the rectal wall toward the back are attached to the vagina, forming a single layer.

If you insert a finger in your vagina, you will feel the bladder in the front, the rectum at the back and the perineal muscles to the sides, including the very powerful levator ani muscle that you can contract on command! Try it out — you will also be testing the tonicity of your vagina.

> **If you insert a finger in your vagina, you will feel the bladder toward the front and the rectum toward the back.**

The Walls of the Bladder, Vagina and Rectum

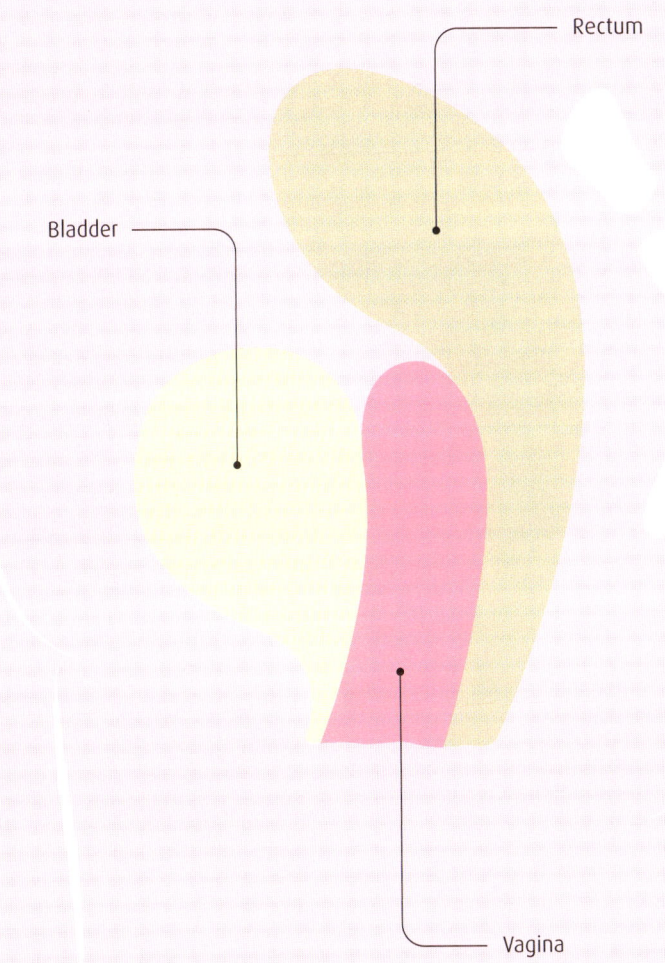

The Vagina in All Its Forms

■ The Vagina in Everyday Life ■

Let's get to know the private life of your vagina. What does it do throughout its cycle? What does it accommodate? How does it expel waste? And finally, what does it do?

What Does It Secrete?

Several factors contribute to vaginal discharge, including vaginal flora, physiologic leukorrhea and cervical mucus. If you are not menopausal or

Having a small amount of whitish discharge is a normal bodily function.

breastfeeding, you will have noticed that your underwear is rarely dry and tends to be lightly stained white at the end of the day — that's normal! The vagina has natural secretions of varying amounts all cycle long. Once a period ends, after a few days or relative dryness, the vulva will feel wet with clear, slimy pre-ovulation cervical mucus. That lasts for three to five days, until ovulation ends. Next comes the cloudy and sticky post-ovulation mucus, and the vulva seems dryer. The week before your next period, a moderate amount of white discharge, which is more liquid than the mucus, reappears.

This description applies only to women with spontaneous

natural cycles — and not those who are taking birth control pills, are pregnant or are menopausal! You can have more or less of a discharge depending on your hormonal state. High levels of estrogen will increase the amount of pre-ovulatory mucus and leukorrhea (normal vaginal discharge). Those who are on the pill will have a moderate amount of discharge, but no ovulatory cervical mucus. Lastly, a menopausal woman will experience more dryness.

First Phase of the Cycle

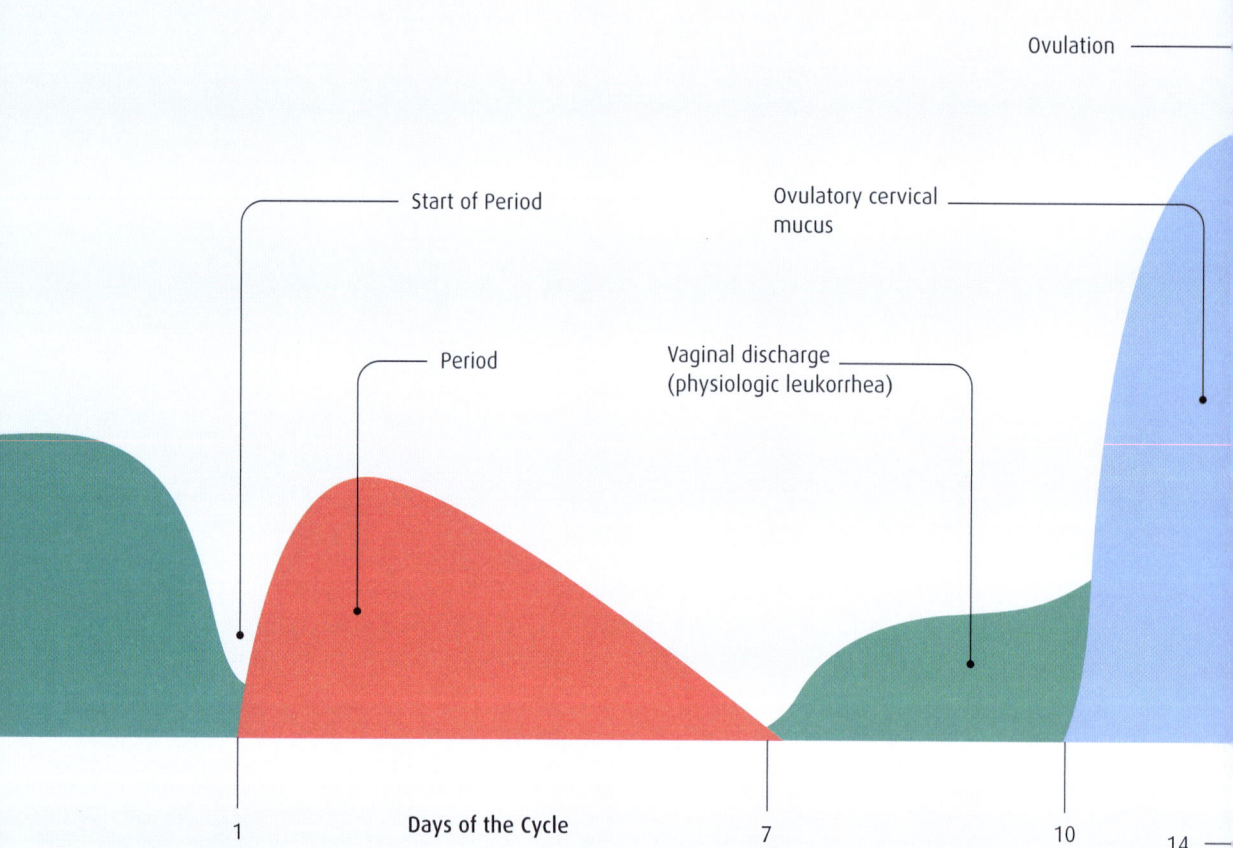

Second Phase of the Cycle

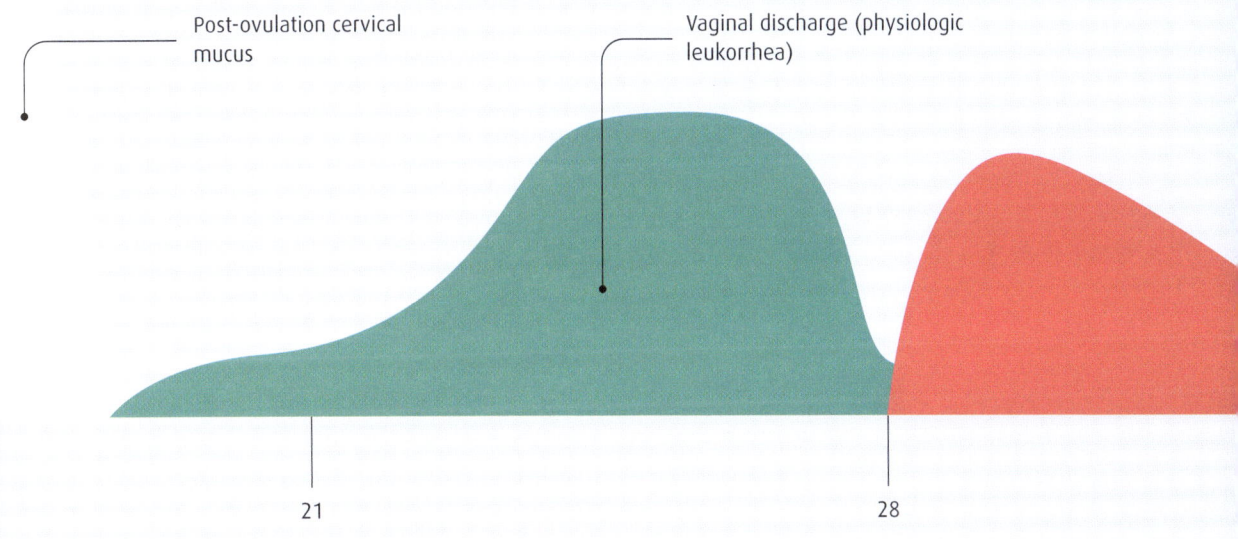

Vaginal Flora

The vagina is an "ecosystem" where, in a healthy female with no gynecological conditions, different types of bacteria live in perfect harmony. The vast majority of bacteria that live naturally in the vaginal flora are the saprophytic bacteria of the *Lactobacillus* genus; they represent 90 percent of the bacteria found in the vagina. Lactobacilli — also called Döderlein's bacilli — are responsible for maintaining the vagina's pH balance, which should fluctuate between 3.8 and 4.5 and is therefore slightly acidic. In comparison, the stomach's pH can drop to 1.5, blood is stable at 7.4 and water has a neutral pH of 7.

Vaginal flora is made up of 90 percent lactobacilli.

Now, back to our tenants! To maintain the vagina's acidity, lactobacilli produce, as the name indicates, lactic acid. These good bacteria, bathing in the acidic juices and vaginal secretions, are behind vaginal discharge. The vaginal ecosystem has a few other "residents" who, in reasonable numbers, are perfectly tolerable. In this melting pot, you will find fungus (e.g. *Candida albicans*); bacteria, including certain bacteria from the stomach (e.g., E. coli) or from the skin (e.g. streptococcus); and small amounts of naturally occurring bacteria in the vagina (e.g., *Gardnerella vaginalis*).

As long as there are enough lactobacilli to ensure an acidic pH, everything is fine. However, beware of disrupting the equilibrium, because the moment a population of bacteria takes over, vulvovaginitis (inflammation of the vulva and vagina) will occur.

Bacteria in the Vagina

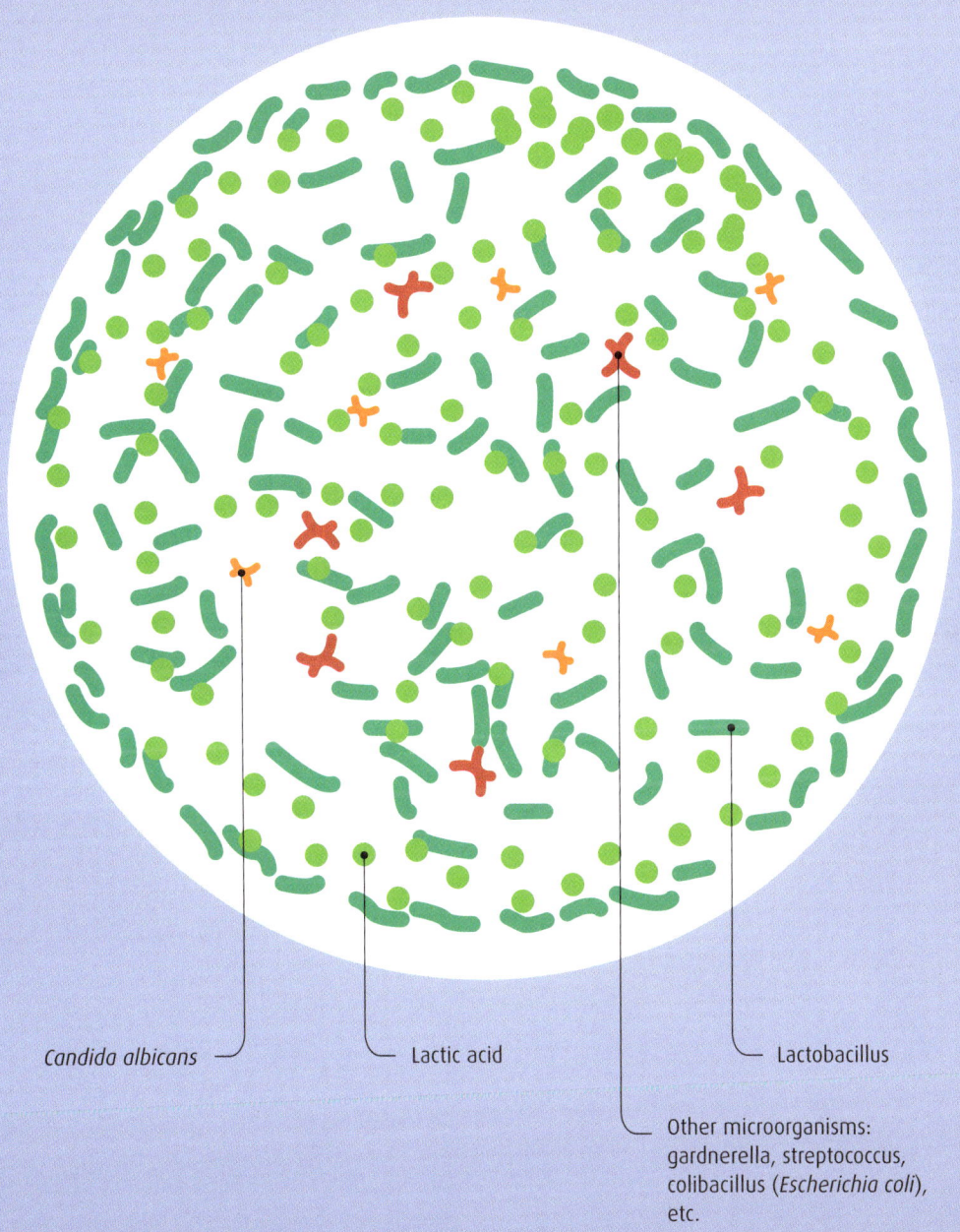

Candida albicans

Lactic acid

Lactobacillus

Other microorganisms: gardnerella, streptococcus, colibacillus (*Escherichia coli*), etc.

Physiologic Leukorrhea

The term "leukorrhea" comes from the Greek words *leuco*, meaning white, and *rhea*, meaning flow. It tells us quite plainly that it's a white flow, and many of you know it as "vaginal discharge." These colorless, painless and odorless discharges naturally mark the phases of the menstrual cycle. Discharge is a liquid made by the vagina and the vaginal bacterial flora. The vagina is covered in a film made up of water and many other substances, including alcohol and glycol complexes. This mucus lines the vaginal walls and is multipurpose. It supports the vagina's immune defense against bacteria and viruses, it eliminates dead cells through "self-cleaning," it promotes the balance of vaginal flora and it helps lubricate during sex. You now understand how important it is to respect this film and, above all, to not strip it by vaginal douching. The vagina is not dirty; it does a great job of cleaning itself!

This mucosal fluid is also called transudate. It is a type of perspiration — in this case, transudation — through thousands of microscopic pores of the vagina's mucus membrane. During sexual arousal, vaginal transudation increases, and, at the time of orgasm, the Skene glands (located near the urethra) release a liquid whose chemical composition is close to that of pre-seminal fluid that precedes ejaculation in males.

> **The vagina is not dirty; it does a great job of cleaning itself!**

Cervical Mucus

In the four or five days before ovulation, the glands in the cervix secrete cervical mucus. During a gynecological exam, with your cervix slightly open using a speculum, your doctor can quite distinctly see this clear and slimy secretion. However, you will notice it (or rather perceive it as feeling "wet") only when it flows out of the vagina. If you are not pregnant, on birth control or menopausal — in other words, if you are ovulating — this discharge is clear like egg whites and stretches between two fingers, feeling stringy and slightly sticky. It is perfectly normal! Cervical mucus indicates the start of a cycle's fertile phase. If you are trying to conceive, you now know what to do and when to do it!

Cervical Mucus

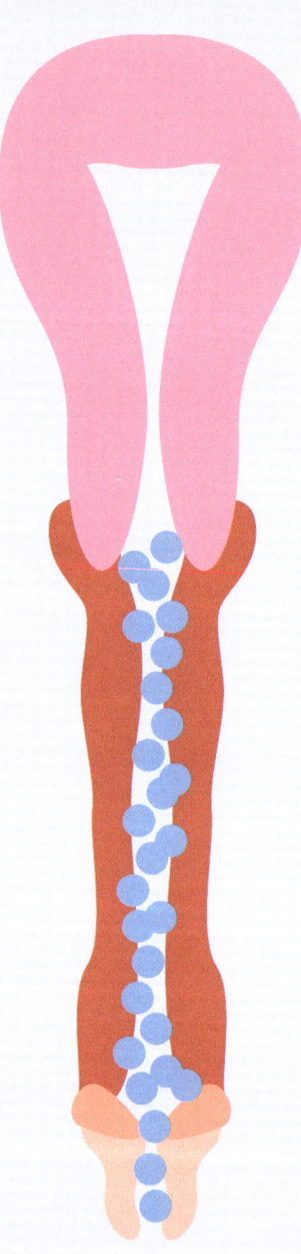

What Is the Vagina For?

The vagina is a passageway, and the flow between the vagina and the uterus, passing through the cervix, is a two-way street.

- From the uterus to the vagina there is the flow of periods and cervical mucus, as well as the passage of a baby during childbirth.

- From the vagina to the uterus, for the purpose of reproduction, there is the deposit of semen deep into the vagina and the upstream swim of determined sperm.

And, of course, don't forget the sensual act of "back and forth" that takes place in the vagina — for the pleasure of both partners.

The Vagina at All Ages

Hormonal changes affect females throughout their lives, every month and throughout their cycle. The vagina also sees significant changes between a young girl, her mother and her grandmother.

From Birth to Puberty

At birth, a baby girl is still full of estrogen from her mother, her vulva is swollen, and there's a milky secretion from the vagina. That dries up very quickly, and the vagina keeps a low profile throughout infancy and until pre-pubescence when, well before the first period, it prepares for its transformation — at the same time breasts and hair start to sprout. The vagina creases, grows and starts transudation. There is, therefore, no reason to stress about the appearance of vaginal discharge in 10-year-old girls, provided that it does not cause irritation, contain pus or have a bad odor.

From Puberty to Menopause: Periods

Once menarche (first period) begins, menstruation sticks around for many years. In the Middle Ages, due to the late age of puberty, several pregnancies and low life expectancy, women would experience around 50 cycles in their lifetime. Today, a woman's biological clock will complete a full 28-day cycle (on average) more than 500 times; she is fertile for about 40 years. That means a 21st-century woman will have a period 10 times more than her 10th-century ancestor!

Having a period should no longer be taboo. We must be able to talk freely about it and, above all, not put our lives on hold during our periods. However, periods are not the only sign of our femininity — far from it! If the amount of menstrual flow, the pain it causes or simply its presence interferes with your freedom, don't hesitate to rid yourself of it. From a medical standpoint, there is no risk in suppressing periods. To do so, there are two options: sustained use of the standard birth control pill or a progesterone pill or an IUD with progesterone.

Periods are not taboo, nor are they the only sign of your femininity!

Menstrual Flow

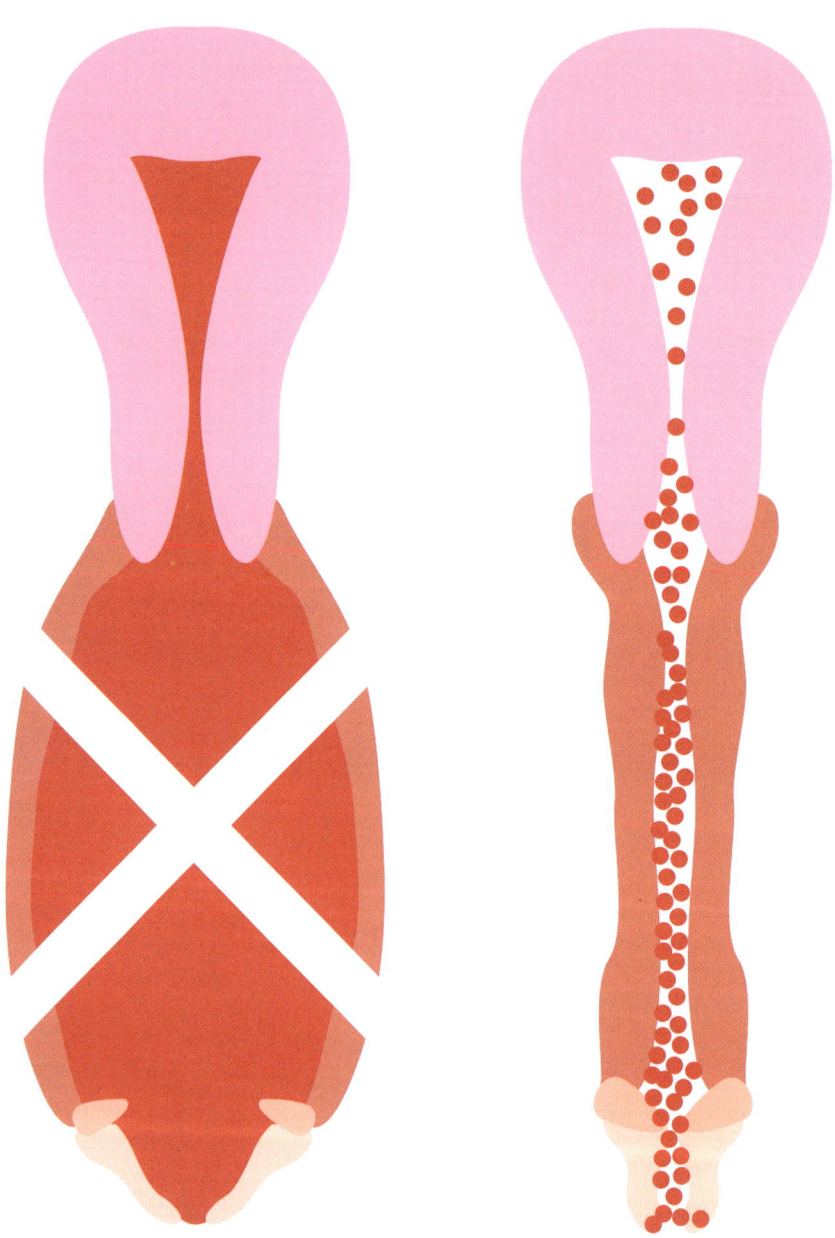

Menstrual Blood

Menstrual blood is not produced by the vagina, but it flows through it. Sometimes, if blood stagnates for a while, it can seem like a certain amount is expelled all at once. Those with perineal muscles that keep the vaginal opening tightly closed can hold blood in their vagina, particularly at night, and let it flow out all at once when they get up. This principle is the basis of "free flow instinct" (also called free instinctive flow). The method relies on the ability to hold blood in the vagina during menstruation and to relax the perineum on demand when on the toilet to empty it. If you listen to the followers of this method, you can also do away with sanitary protection without the risk of staining your underwear. I don't recommend that you try that if you have a heavy flow and are wearing white pants, but this ecologically and economically sound technique could make sense for moderate bleeding — and in the comfort of your own home.

If you have a heavy flow and it remains in your vagina, blood clots can form. They are nothing to worry about, unless it's a sign of menorrhagia (heavy menstrual bleeding), which is a different matter. On the other hand, a small amount of blood

> **The vagina plays a part in the look and smell of your period.**

that pools in the vagina becomes a brown discharge, sometimes very dark, that looks like sand when it dries. Again, there is no need to worry! The vagina plays a part in both the look and smell of your period. Indeed, the stagnation of blood in the vagina, be it through long and heavy periods or spotting (small continuous bleeding), can be the cause of change in vaginal flora called vaginosis.

The Menstrual Cycle

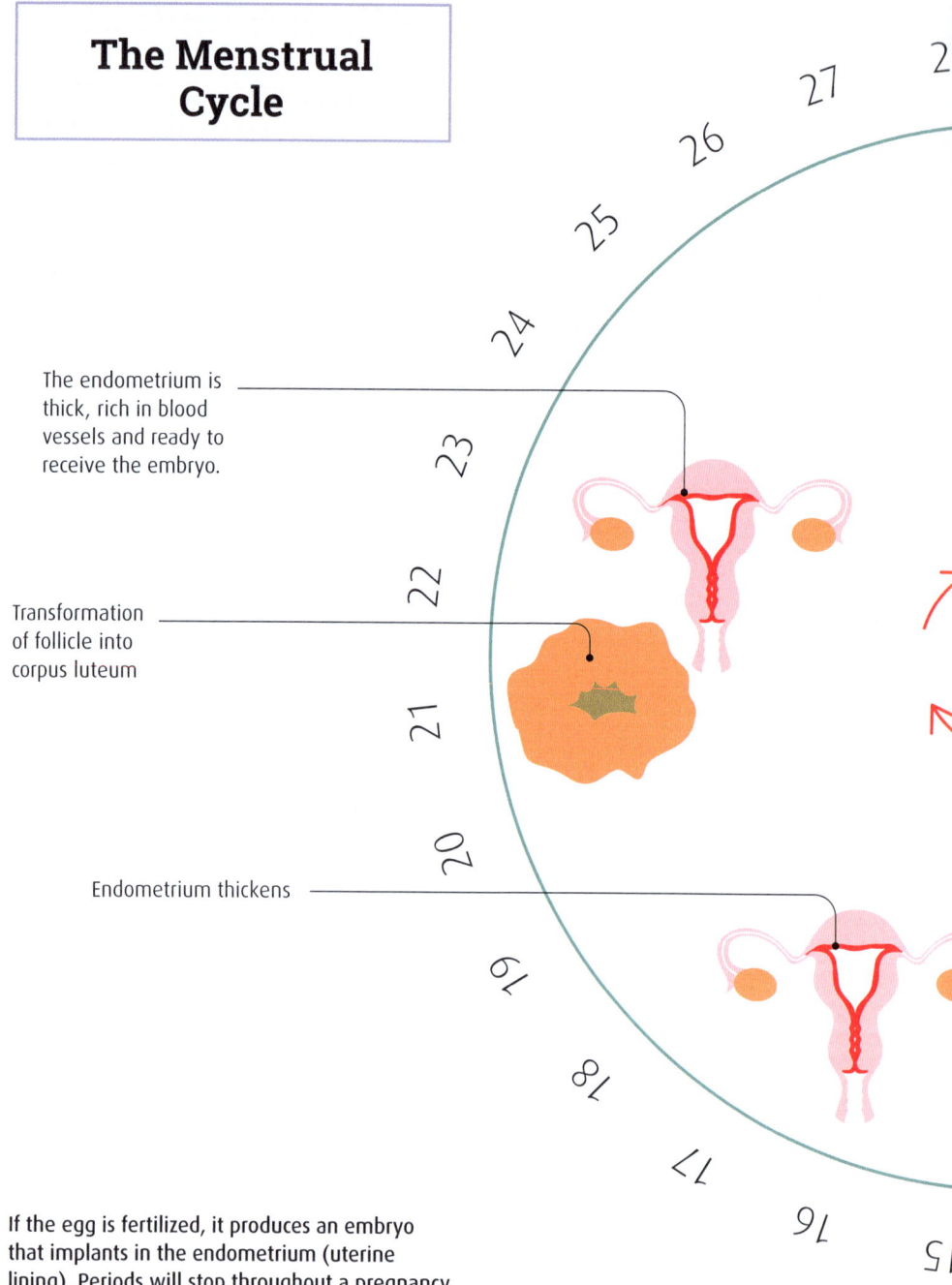

The endometrium is thick, rich in blood vessels and ready to receive the embryo.

Transformation of follicle into corpus luteum

Endometrium thickens

If the egg is fertilized, it produces an embryo that implants in the endometrium (uterine lining). Periods will stop throughout a pregnancy.

If the egg is not fertilized, the cycle restarts.

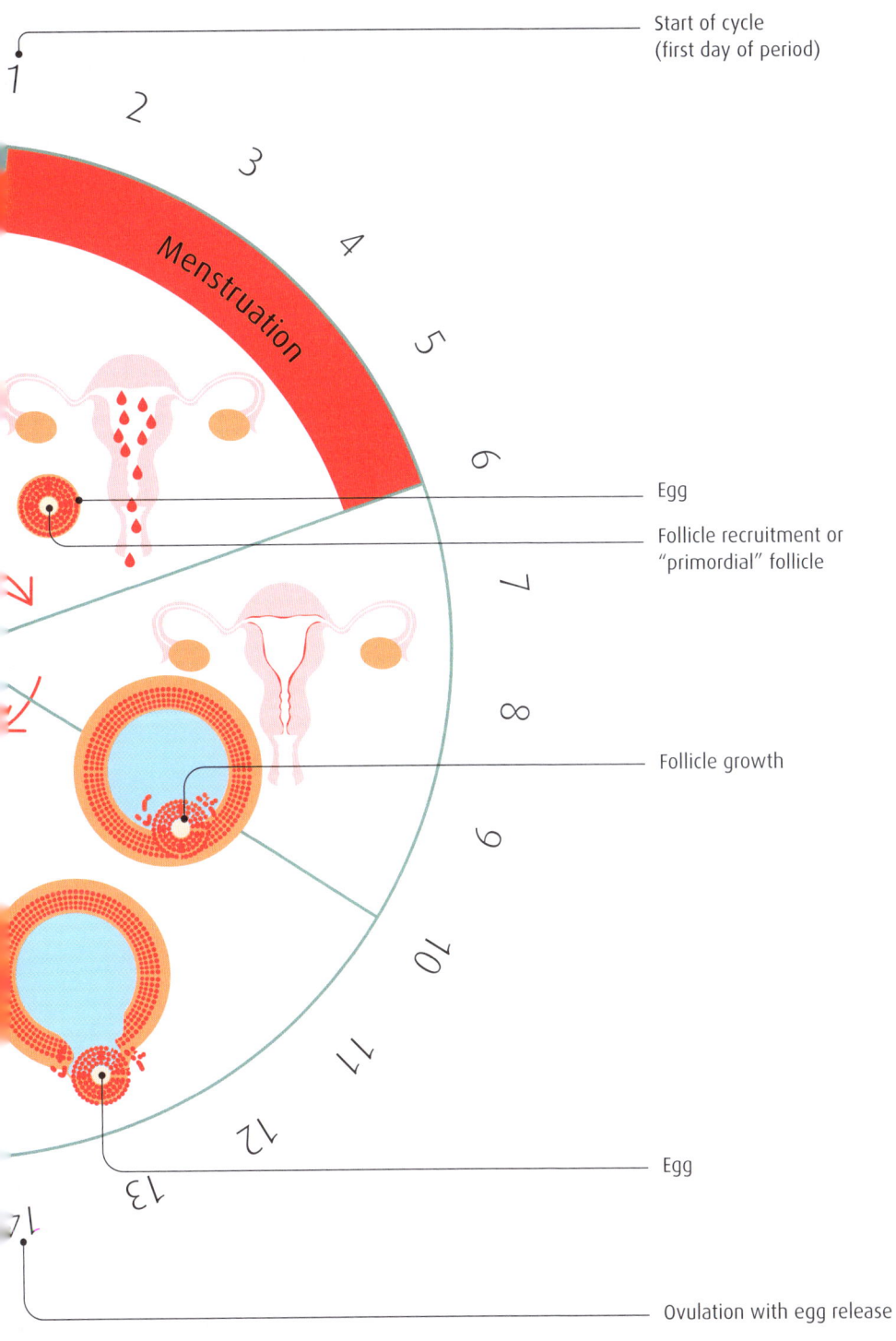

Tampons

First, I would like to encourage you to use feminine hygiene products that you insert inside the vagina rather than sanitary napkins (pads). A young girl who can insert a tampon will never suffer from vaginismus.

> **Toxic Shock Syndrome stems from leaving in a tampon for an extended period of time.**

Knowing your vagina is always an advantage. Feeling free to swim or wear a thong – that's even better!

Tampons, however, get some bad press; they are blamed for causing staphylococcal toxic shock syndrome (TSS) and contain potentially toxic materials. TSS is rare (according to one recent study, the incidence of TSS in the United States is 0.8 to 3.4 per 100,000.) but serious. This infection, linked to a toxin in staphylococcus bacteria, occurs only during menstruation. It is further facilitated by the prolonged use (more than four hours) of a tampon or menstrual cup (even rarer from use of a pad). Copper IUDs and the use of a menstrual cup slightly raise the risk. However, of the millions of tampons used in North America every year, TSS does not occur often. TSS mostly affects young women between the ages of 14 and 24 who are healthy carriers of staphylococcus (around 20 percent of the population carries this bacterium in their nasal cavities, on their skin or in their vagina with no effect on their health). Symptoms include a high fever, a peeling rash, extreme dizziness with low blood pressure, diarrhea and vomiting. It is a medical emergency that requires intensive care and hospitalization.

Tampons are also not environmentally friendly and create a lot of waste. Some bleaching, softening and antibacterial products that are used in the manufacturing of tampons are suspected of being endocrine disrupters — whose absorption through the vaginal walls is quite significant.

Endocrine disruptors are chemical or natural substances that, even in small amounts, interfere with the endocrine system by imitating hormones, particularly sex and thyroid hormones. They are found just about everywhere in the environment. The exposure to endocrine disruptors is more dangerous during pregnancy (for the fetus) and early childhood. They are associated with urogenital defects in male infants (cryptorchidism and hypospadias), psycho-behavioral developmental disorders (hyperactivity and autism spectrum disorder), early-onset puberty and male and female infertility.

The Endocrine System: Our Body's Key Regulator

- Hypothalamus
- Hypophysis (pituitary gland)
- Thyroid
- Thymus
- Pancreas
- Adrenal glands
- Ovaries

The endocrine system regulates several bodily functions like growth, behavior, reproduction and stress management.

Menstrual Cups

From an environmental standpoint, a menstrual cup is, without a doubt, better than tampons or pads. However, make sure you choose the material of your cup carefully: opt for a pharmaceutical brand that uses medical-grade silicone. With a starting investment of around $20, this device has the advantage of being affordable. It creates no waste and is economical since you can reuse it many times after a simple sterilization in boiling water. It's comfortable, as long as you choose the right size to prevent leaks and avoid irritation from the stem touching your labia.

You will need a little more dexterity to insert a cup than you would for a tampon. A complete seal is not guaranteed, especially during the learning period. It is, therefore, recommended that you get comfortable with the sight of blood and make sure there is a sink nearby. If you have an IUD, do not pull the cup out directly; instead, grip and pinch the cup first to avoid a suction-cup effect.

Don't go so far with any zero-waste initiatives as to acquire or buy a used cup. Even if it's boiled, there is still a risk of transmission of certain viruses. However, sterilizing your own cup with boiling water is largely sufficient. Think about sterilizing it at the end of every period and before putting it back in its case.

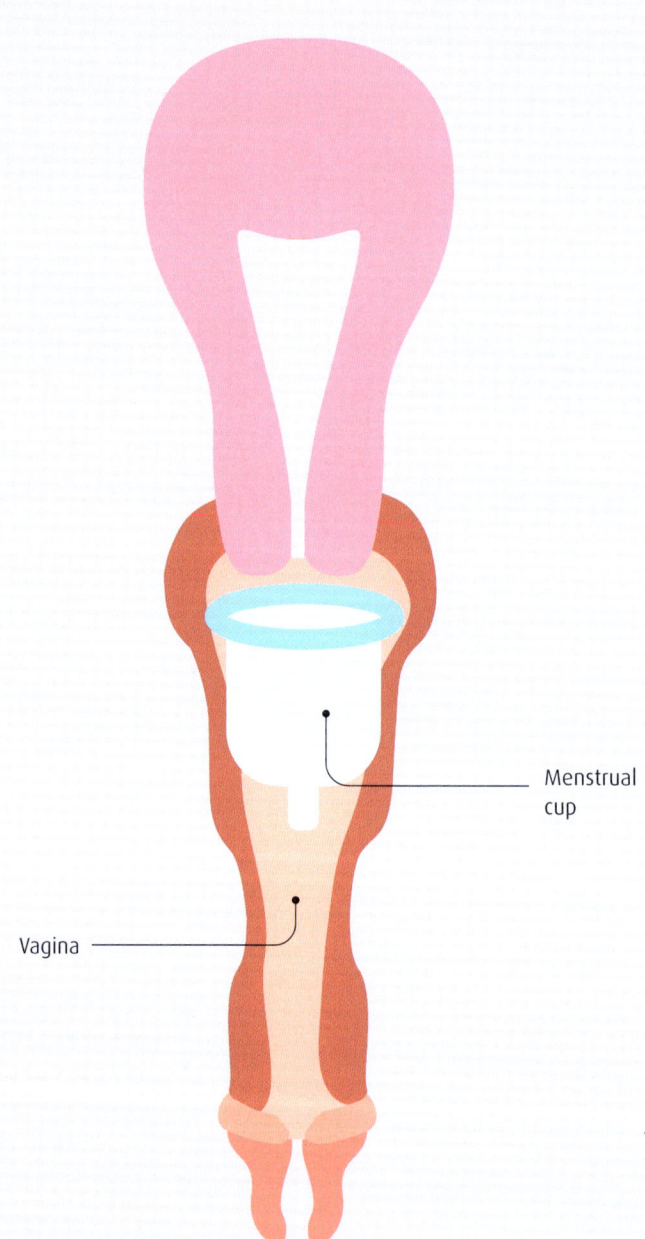

Hormone Therapy

In cases of menorrhagia (heavy menstrual bleeding); mastodynia (breast pain); certain conditions, like endometriosis; and benign tumors, like fibroids, your gynecologist may prescribe a progestogen to block your cycle. Some progestogen medications in the norpregnane family drastically reduce your estrogen levels. That's good for your breasts and your periods, but terrible for your vaginal secretions. In the case of vaginal dryness, you will need to take an estrogen supplement — usually administered systemically as, in the long run, vaginally is too inconvenient. The challenge will be to find the correct dosage to "punch up" your vaginal mucosa without overriding the therapeutic effect of your progestogen medication.

Menopause

Estrogen is a hormone that regulates and nourishes our vaginal mucosa and helps to maintain vaginal flora. When menopause starts, estrogen becomes scarce. Vaginal mucosa without estrogen is like a pair of luxury shoes that you never polish. It loses its luster and flexibility and cracks. The mucosa changes: its slightly wrinkly appearance becomes smoother; its color turns from pinkish red to pearly pink; and fine, small vessels sometimes rise to the surface, to the point where the slightest touch makes them bleed. Secretions have almost entirely dried up — it's the start of the great drought!

> **A menopausal woman with a regular sex life will have good-quality vaginal mucosa.**

You might be asking yourself "Is this unavoidable?" Luckily, no. The vagina works opposite to a battery: It will wear out if it's not being used! In other words, a menopausal woman (even one who has been menopausal for a long time) who maintains a regular sex life will have good-quality vaginal mucosa. When it comes to desire, in a strictly hormonal sense, it will have every reason to improve. In fact, if the ovaries don't produce more estrogen, the adrenal glands (located above the kidneys) will, in turn, continue to produce the male hormone testosterone. Great for your libido, but not so great for your facial hair — you can't have everything!

However, if your sex life is struggling before menopause, don't expect a miracle! An Australian study[1] has shown that the quality of a woman's sex life during menopause is correlated with prior sexual satisfaction and, of

---

1. L. Dennerstein, P. Lehert, and H. Burger, "The Relative Effects of Hormones and Relationship Factors on Sexual Function of Women Through the Natural Menopausal Transition," *Fertil Steril*, 84 (July 2005): 174–80.

course, dependent on the relationship between partners.

Menopausal hormone therapy (MHT) can counter the inconveniences caused by a lack of estrogen, including vaginal dryness. Since it provides estrogen, menopausal hormone therapy will always be beneficial for vaginal mucosa — helping to maintain hydration, elasticity and lubrication from sexual stimulation and reducing the risk of vaginal and urinary infections.

If you cannot or do not want to take MHT, it is possible to treat the vagina locally with estrogen in the form of creams, tablets or slow-release vaginal rings that last for three months. If a local treatment is not possible or desired, other options include hydrophilic or hyaluronic acid gels that can be applied three times a week with a single-dose applicator. However, I have noticed that, over time, due to costs and limitations, women tend to get tired of taking such treatments.

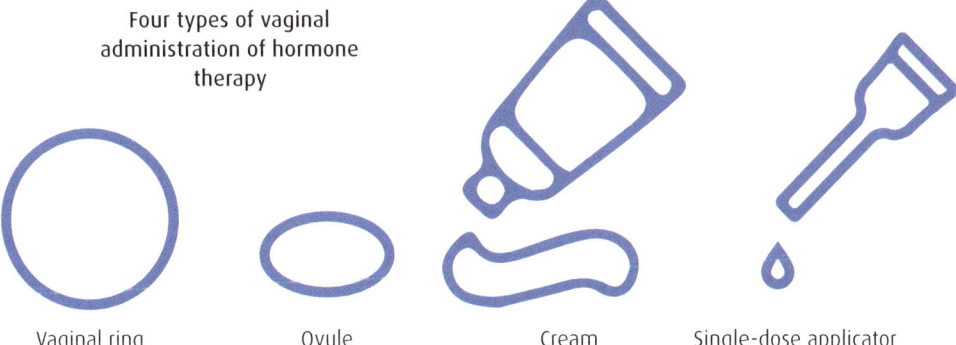

Four types of vaginal administration of hormone therapy

Vaginal ring — Ovule — Cream — Single-dose applicator

To thicken vaginal mucosa, alleviate dryness and restart the vagina's ability to lubricate itself, endovaginal laser treatment can be a big help. Note, however, that if your vagina has been dormant for a while, with no prospect of reigniting sexual activity, it's a waste of money! However, endovaginal laser seems to me like a very good option for women taking adjuvant therapy (aromatase inhibitors) as a result of hormone-dependent breast cancer. In fact, all local and systemic estrogen treatments are contraindicated for those patients, but for those who had a satisfying sex life prior to their illness, laser therapy can at least provide vaginal comfort.

Like the vagina, the rest of the female genitalia is not immune to the ravages of time. As for aging skin and subcutaneous tissue, there is a loss of elasticity and a decrease in the supportive connective tissue of the hypodermis. Does that ring any bells? Wrinkles! The same goes for the labia majora and labia minora, which start to sag. For those who can't bare these entirely natural changes, know that even for this body part, there are interesting esthetic medical solutions, like hyaluronic acid injections. These injections can also help manage pain caused by vestibule fragility during sex.

We are neither robots nor animals, and your sex life is more than body parts, hormones and mucus. Menopause marks an important stage in a woman's sex life. Changes related to menopause, as well as age or certain conditions affecting your partner or partners, require some adjustments. Even if you have a deep desire, your vagina will likely be a bit slow to start, so you will need to take your time. As for any male partners you may have, if they are around the same age as you, they will also have aging arteries, so their erection will be more fragile and they may not be able to wait for you. Regardless, it won't help the matter if your partner thinks you are not really interested or if they lose confidence in their ability to make you orgasm.

So there's only one thing to do: communicate! Explain that you are simply low on fuel and need a longer warm-up period (most people understand perfectly well what that means). To shorten

Lube helps jump-start your own vaginal lubrication.

this "warm-up," don't hesitate to use lube. Caresses will be more enjoyable and arousal will be heightened, which stimulates the vaginal lubrication and helps it quickly reach the vestibule. Penetration can thereby happen more quickly and will be painless.

The Vagina and New Life

From conception through pregnancy, childbirth and breastfeeding, what a roller coaster for your vagina!

Conception

Collecting sperm to conceive a baby — here is yet another key function of the vagina. Sperm is deposited deep in the vagina in the posterior fornix. There, it comes in contact with the cervical mucus, in which sperm are more mobile and agile — skills that are essential for traveling from the cervix to the uterus and finally into one of the fallopian tubes. This journey, worthy of an expert swimmer, has only one purpose: to meet and fertilize the egg. What a mission! For a microscopic sperm, that's like swimming across the ocean, and as you know, only one will make it.

There are only three or four truly fertile days within a cycle, so don't miss them. To know which days you're fertile, take note of your cervical mucus, which, around day 10 of a 28-day cycle, will appear slippery, stretchy and clear like egg whites. If, from one day to the next, the vulva is drier and the discharge is cloudy and sticky, that means the fertile period is over. All that's left to do is hope you've gotten pregnant or wait for the next cycle.

> **There are only 3 or 4 truly fertile days in a cycle.**

Pregnancy

When a woman is pregnant, she is literally pumped with estrogen, the ultimate female hormone. Her vaginal mucosa is better for it because the secretions are more abundant. Frequent vaginal discharge throughout the pregnancy is nothing to worry about. However, if you notice a very liquidy, water-like discharge, it could be the amniotic fluid, a sign that you should head to the hospital right away.

Childbirth

The transformation of the vagina at childbirth is absolutely amazing. The cervix disappears! Yes, you read that right. The uterus and the vagina form a single passage for the baby to make his or her way through.

Breastfeeding

Hormonal changes that happen when nursing, particularly the secretion of prolactin, are responsible for vaginal dryness. It is important to educate young mothers about this because oftentimes there is apprehension about returning to their sex life. My advice: educate the young father too, relax and use lube.

The Vagina During Childbirth

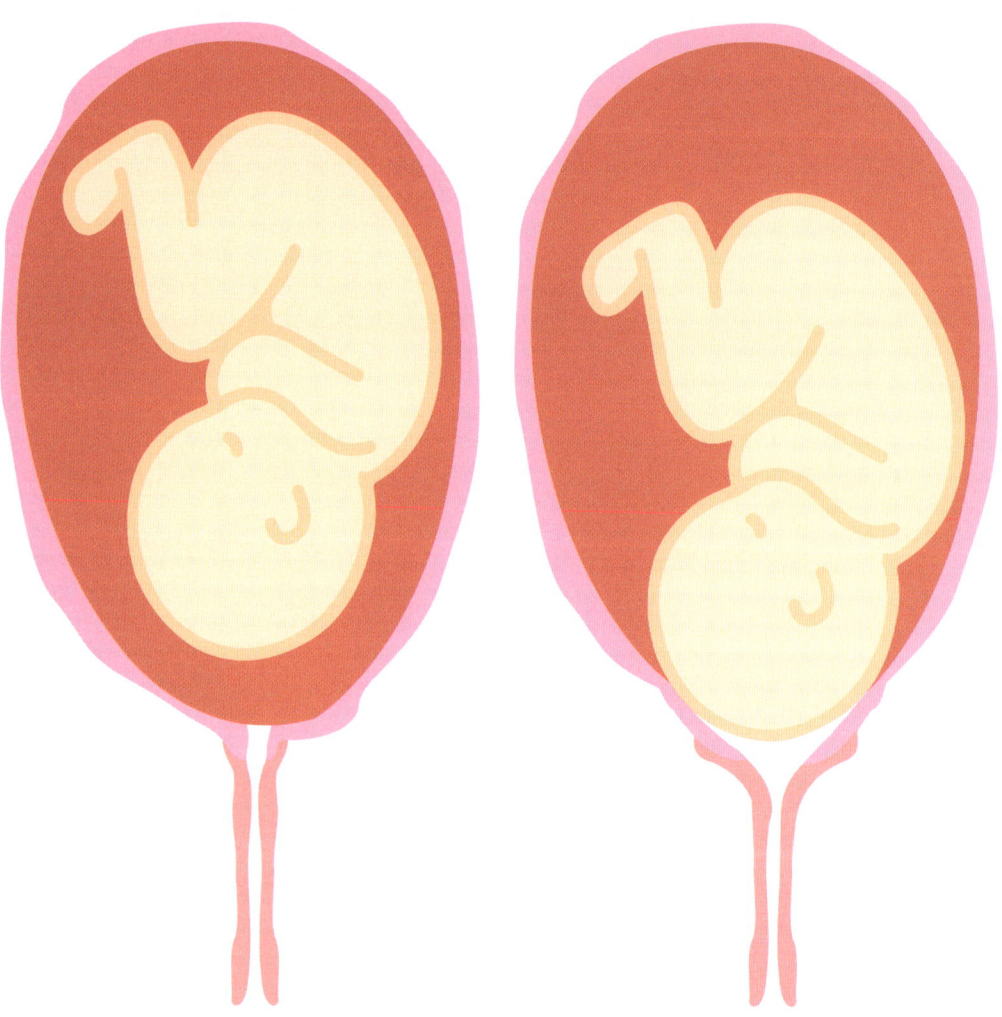

During pregnancy, the uterus and vagina are separated by the cervix.

During labor, the cervix shrinks and opens.

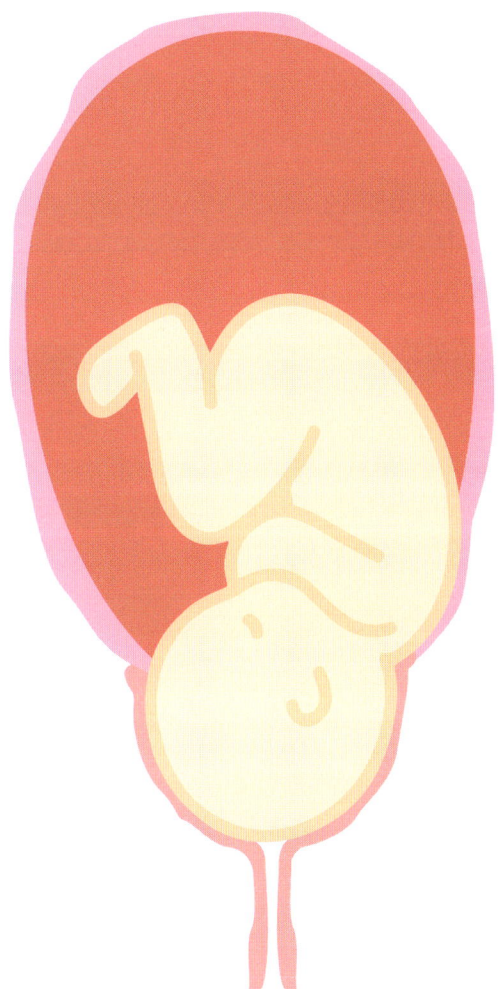

During delivery, the uterus and the vagina become one, and the cervix disappears.

The Vagina for Pleasure!

There is always much curiosity about pleasure associated with the vagina and orgasm. Read on for the latest information!

Vaginal Lubrication

Before reaching orgasm, dear reader, you must go back to square one: "arousal" and lubrication, which go hand in hand. Your main sex organ is your brain, the source of desires and fantasies. Under the very particular and special circumstances of sex, your brain throws reason and etiquette out the window, so you feel uninhibited and do things you might otherwise consider contrary to good manners.

An erotic image or thought are powerful enough to initiate lubrication before foreplay even begins. Since lubrication mainly comes from the transudation of walls deep within the vagina, it will be some time before you and your partner will notice it in the vaginal opening. During foreplay, arousal of the main erogenous zones — her majesty the clitoris first in line, followed by breasts, hair, inner thighs and so on — will finish what your imagination started. The amount and appearance of vaginal lubrication at the vulva is proportional to the intensity of arousal and the responsiveness of the vaginal mucosa.

This lubrication's ability to actually lubricate depends on its thickness and the estrogen levels. For that reason, under certain conditions

> **Lubrication depends as much on arousal as on vaginal responsiveness.**

like menopause, some breast cancer treatments and radiation, lubrication is sometimes a challenge.

Vaginal Orgasm

At the risk of deceiving you, the true vaginal orgasm, after some minutes of back and forth, happens once in a blue moon — and still I am optimistic! Orgasms are mainly clitoral, and the best way to climax is to use both penetration and clitoral stimulation. Outside of the bottom quarter of the vagina, the part closest to the vestibule and the famous G spot, the vagina itself is not very sensitive. You can feel your bladder when its full, your rectum when you have to go to the bathroom, your stomach when you feel hungry — but radio silence from your vagina! When the vagina is penetrated, you will experience a deep, overall sensation, but three-quarters of your vagina will feel neither pain nor pleasure. The cervix, particularly the cervical canal, belongs to another sensitive system that will undoubtedly send you a pain signal if something brushes against, for example when inserting an IUD.

> **The clitoris helps you orgasm more often and more easily than the vagina.**

How Does an Orgasm Work?

3
Orgasm
Duration: Several seconds

2
Plateau
Duration: From a few seconds to several minutes

1
Arousal
Duration: From a few minutes to several hours

The Vagina for Pleasure! | 59

Usual orgasm peak

Double orgasm (rare!)

No orgasm

4

Resolution
Duration: Generally a few minutes

What About the G Spot?

It's not a myth. The G spot is an anatomical and functional reality, but do not expect too much from it all the same. It is in no way the on/off button for the vaginal orgasm. Furthermore, it did not come out of nowhere, but from observations by a very serious German gynecologist, Doctor Ernst Gräfenberg, who described it in 1950 as a zone on the front vaginal wall, close to the urethra (the canal that carries urine from the bladder outward). It wasn't until 30 years later, when it was named the Gräfenberg spot, that its popularity increased! Since then, debates and studies have taken place to confirm its existence, to locate it (with ultrasounds and MRIs) and, above all, to understand how it works. For some, it is closely connected to the deep-lying parts of the clitoris. That's why the orgasm is an overall vaginal and clitoral reaction.

The proximity of the G spot to the urinary system is an important fact because its stimulation can result in the urge to urinate. The term "spot" is perhaps not the best fit; it is not a spot but rather a zone, the size of a quarter, located on the front vaginal wall (the bladder side), about 1½ inches (4 cm) from the vaginal opening. To find it, insert a finger into your vagina up to the second joint, bend the finger toward the front side of the vaginal wall and feel around. Outside of a sexual arousal context, you will feel only a slight urge to pee.

The G spot does not automatically trigger a vaginal orgasm!

During an orgasm, this zone, rich in nerves and blood vessels, is able to swell and secrete a large quantity of fluid thanks to the Skene glands. The G spot is one of the mechanisms cited to explain the phenomenon of female ejaculation. Its splendor is presumed to be within reach of every woman — provided you can find it and know how to stimulate it. That's all very well, you might say, but does its stimulation guarantee an ascent to cloud nine at the speed of light? Absolutely not. The organ whose only and noble purpose is exclusively for pleasure is not the G spot but the clitoris. Vaginal-only orgasms are rare, occurring for less than 20 percent of women. However, sexual arousal of both the clitoris and vagina – in particularly the G spot – gets 5 gold stars for pleasure. Bravo, vagina!

G Spot, Where Are You?
(sectional view)

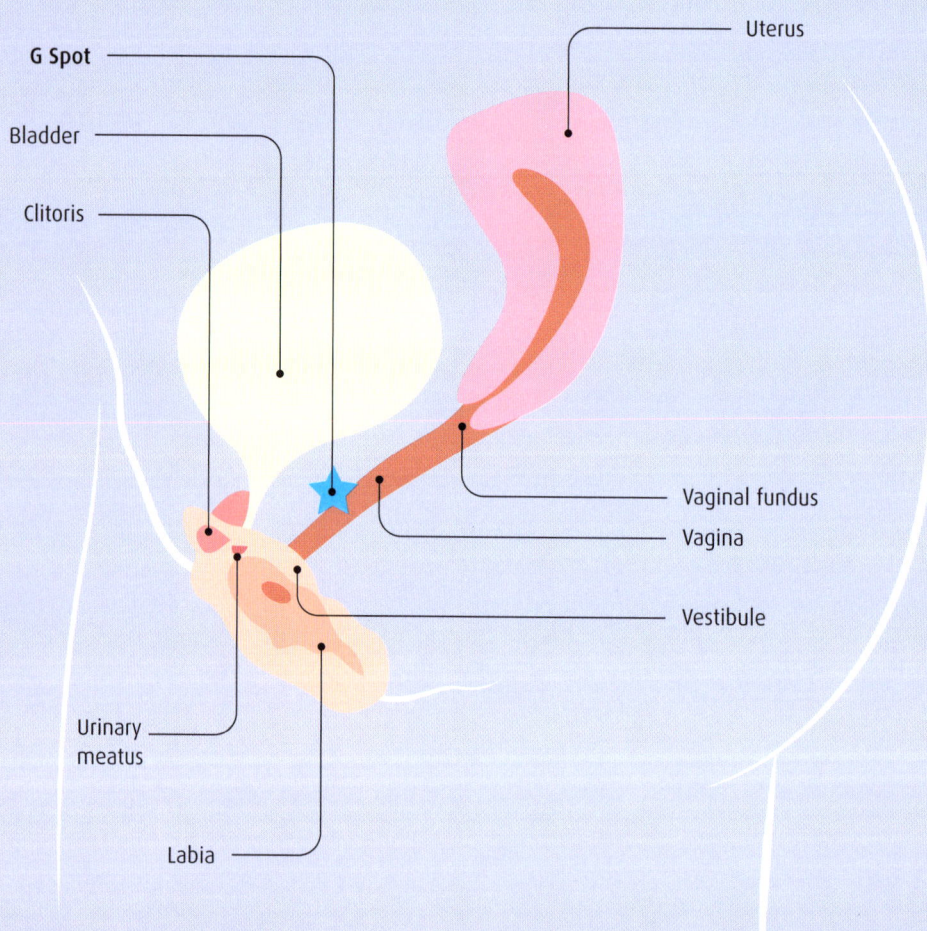

Sex Toys

Did you know that dildos have been around since antiquity? They are called *olisbos* in ancient Greek which translates to "leather penis." The Latin term for dildo, *gaude mihi*, means "give me pleasure."— much more explicit! Erect penises have also been found in frescoes and sculptures among prehistoric remains. That does not, however, mean that they were used by Mrs. Cro-Magnon for, well, you know. Today, dildos are available in a range of sizes, colors and scents and can be purchased in stores and online. They all claim to stimulate your G spot. With the advent of electricity (among other things) came the vibrator. But remember, we just discussed that this zone cannot automatically set off an orgasm. Among the more advanced models, the "Rabbit" dildo has two small "ears" that stimulate the clitoris while the main part of the device enters the vagina and arouses the G spot. Vibrating underwear are also available, which can be used discretely.

> **The Latin term for dildo, *gaude mihi*, means "give me pleasure."**

In ancient times, sailors and soldiers would leave dildos for their wives so they wouldn't get bored — interpret that as you will — or go off with a young wanderer passing through.[2] Still better than a chastity belt, wouldn't you say?

With global sales upward of $23 billion per year, sex toys have become an everyday item found in the nightstand of many women and couples. Today, they're not just used by women

---

2. Gilles Delluc and Brigitte Delluc, "Le Sexe au temps des Cro-Magnons," *Pilote* 24, cited by Emmanuelle Peyret in "Godes antiques," *Libération* (July 2012).

in a sexual dry spell; they also help you explore and discover your vagina's sensuality and, if you're game, to spice up your relationship. Remember: always clean your sex toy, never borrow or lend out a sex toy and, unless stated otherwise by the manufacturer, do not use it under water.

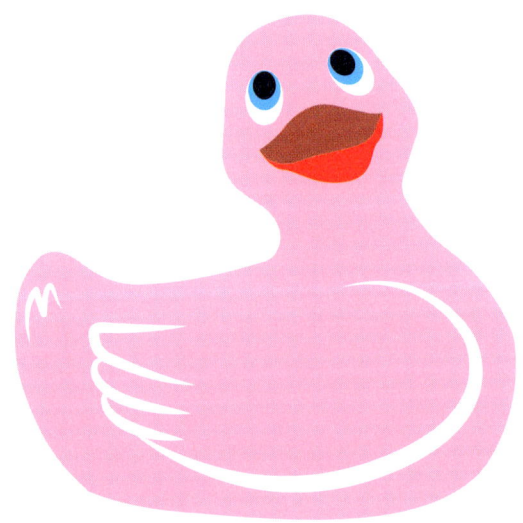

Vaginal Flatulence

This phenomenon, which is uncommon but very embarrassing as it has the tendency to happen during sex, is the result of trapped air in the vagina. When moving or relaxing the perineum, a small amount of air enters the vagina. Because the perineum is tonic, the vagina closes, locking in air until… it escapes and makes a sound. Completely odorless, vaginal flatulence has nothing to do with its digestive counterpart. If you are prone to this gynecological gaffe, squat down, relax your perineum, insert your thumb into the vagina while pressing downward and then squeeze the perineum while gradually removing your thumb. You can use the same technique to remove sperm for the vagina after sex. It's not very glamorous, but it works!

Vaginal flatulence is caused by trapped air in the vagina.

The Vagina and Contraceptives

There are all sorts of contraceptives. From all the options, there are two main types: contraceptives that prevent ovulation (pill, ring, implant) and contraceptives that comply with the menstrual cycle (IUDs, condoms).

The first type, because they change the hormonal balance, can affect the vaginal physiology. The second type interfere very little with the functioning of the vagina. It's up to you to find the one that works best for you!

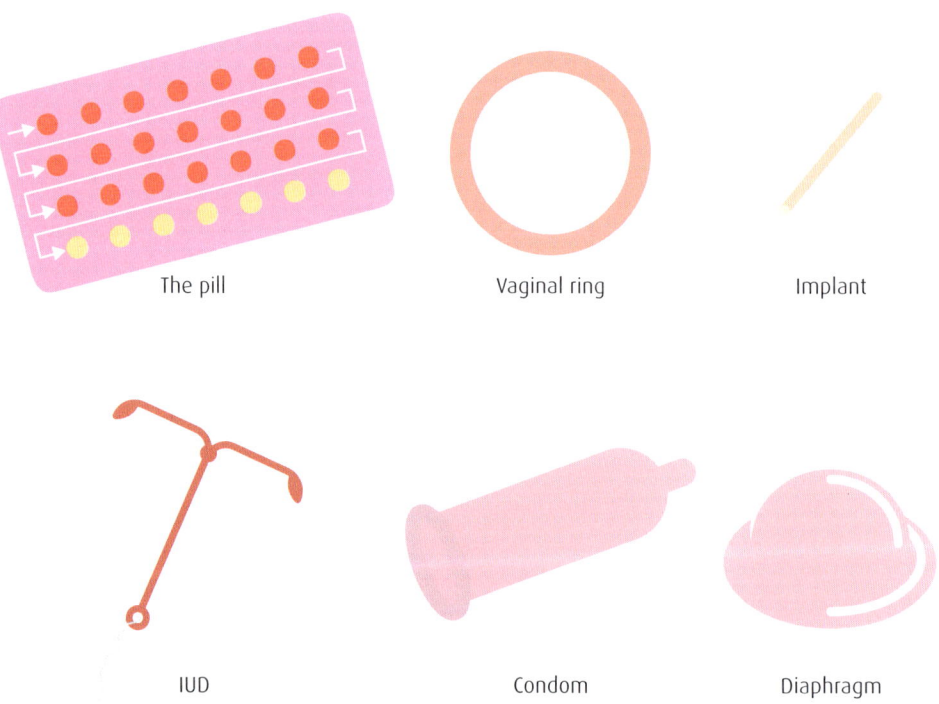

The pill · Vaginal ring · Implant

IUD · Condom · Diaphragm

The Pill

Is the vagina drier when you're on the pill? The answer is: it depends. Because the pill prevents ovulation, logically you will not see any cervical mucus. As for vaginal discharge, there is generally less discharge if there is a lower dosage of estrogen in the pill. The same principle applies for periods: less estrogen, fewer periods!

Nowadays, only mini-pills are sold. The term "mini" refers to the dosage of estrogen, which ranges from 15 to 35 ng (nanograms). As the first course of treatment, you will be prescribed second-generation birth control pills with a dosage of 20 ng of estrogen. They are just as effective as pills with higher quantities of estrogen, and the vascular risk with second-generation progestogen is lower than that with third-generation pills.

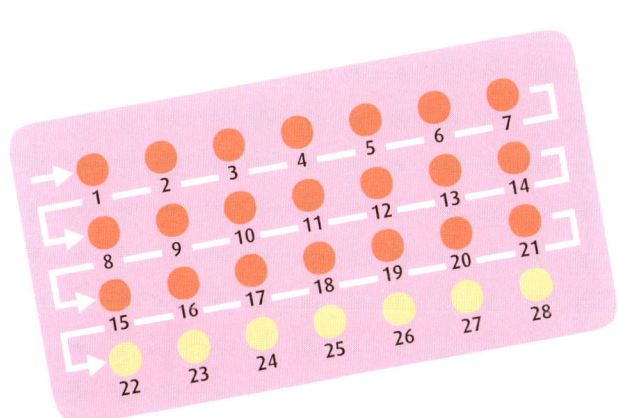

Vaginal Rings

The composition of a vaginal ring is no different than that of the traditional pill, but the hormones are released directly into the vagina and not administered orally. The ring (just like contraceptive implants) is made of a special material (hormone molecules are key) and very convenient, capable of releasing small quantities of hormones over a long period of time. Thanks to this local delivery of estrogen, the vaginal ring has a beneficial effect on vaginal flora. Any woman who knows how to insert a tampon without an applicator can put in a vaginal ring.

Held in place by the vaginal walls, this intravaginal device will go unnoticed by you and your partner. Vaginal mucosa is permeable to several substances, so it's one possible way to administer certain medications. It prevents what's called first-pass metabolism, and the molecules thereby pass directly into the bloodstream. When taken orally, these substances must first pass through the digestive system and then be transformed by the liver before they can start working. Vaginal administration can improve tolerance and decrease side effects inherent to certain treatments.

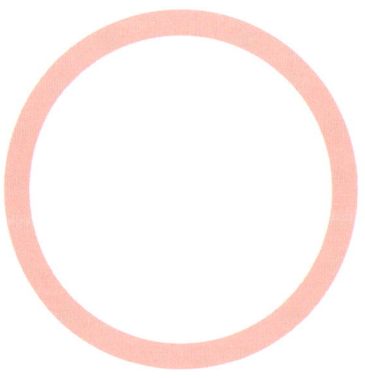

Placement of a Vaginal Ring

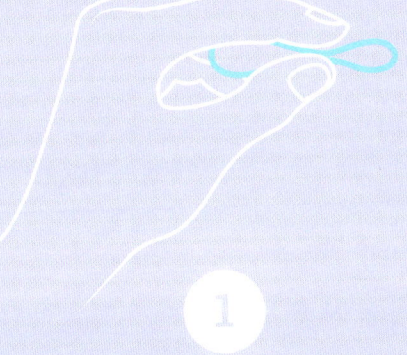

1

Hold the ring between your thumb finger and index.

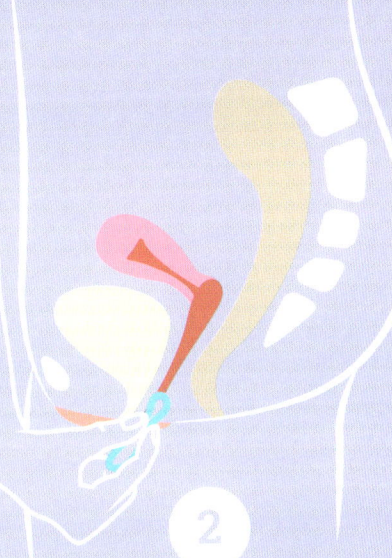

2

Insert the ring into your vagina.

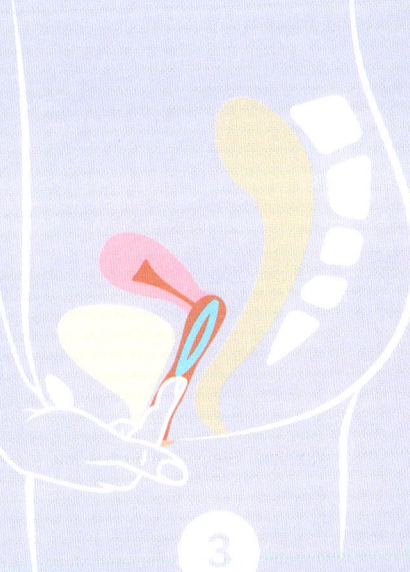

3

Push the ring with your index finger into position.

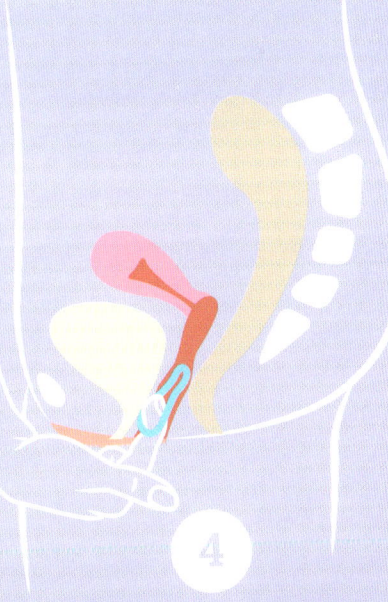

4

To remove the ring, hook it with your index finger and pull.

Desogestrel Implants and Pills

These progestogen-only contraceptives have a unique bleeding profile: either they cause amenorrhea (complete absence of periods) or constant or more frequent spotting. About 30 to 50 percent of women with an implant still bleed, but it is uncommon with desogestrel pills. Women may also experience vaginal dryness due to the lack of estrogen in these contraceptives. If you are one of the women who still bleeds, the pH of your vagina will increase, which may lead to an imbalance in your flora, causing bacterial vaginosis with foul-smelling vaginal discharge.

> **30 to 50 percent of women with a desogestrel implant still bleed, but it is uncommon with desogestrel pills.**

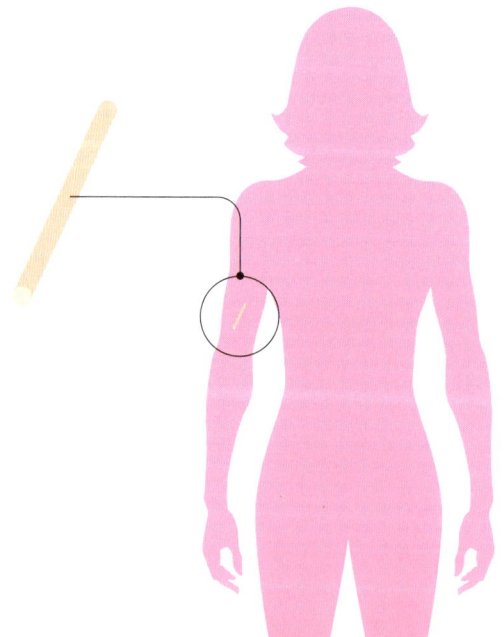

IUDs

All IUDs, whether copper or progesterone, are inserted in the uterus, completely inaccessible to you and your partner. By putting a finger in your vagina, you will feel a nylon string, somewhat rigid like fishing line, poking out of your cervix. After your period, it's important to check that it's still there, even though IUD expulsion is rare. If the string is still the same length, that means the IUD has remained in place. However, if the string seems much longer, it's possible that the IUD has moved, which requires attention from the health-care provider who inserted it. Some gynecologists leave the string hanging a bit longer, while others leave it shorter — it's up to you to ask about it.

Rest assured, there is no risk if it brushes against underwear, but your partner might complain about feeling the thread. If that happens, all you need to do is tuck it in so that it doesn't pass the cervix. The only downside is that you will have to fish for the IUD when it's time for removal, which can be a bit difficult.

For those who use a menstrual cup, be careful if you have an IUD. The suction effect of the cup can potentially move your IUD. To prevent that, put a finger between the cup and the cervix when you pull it out.

Placement of an IUD in the Uterus

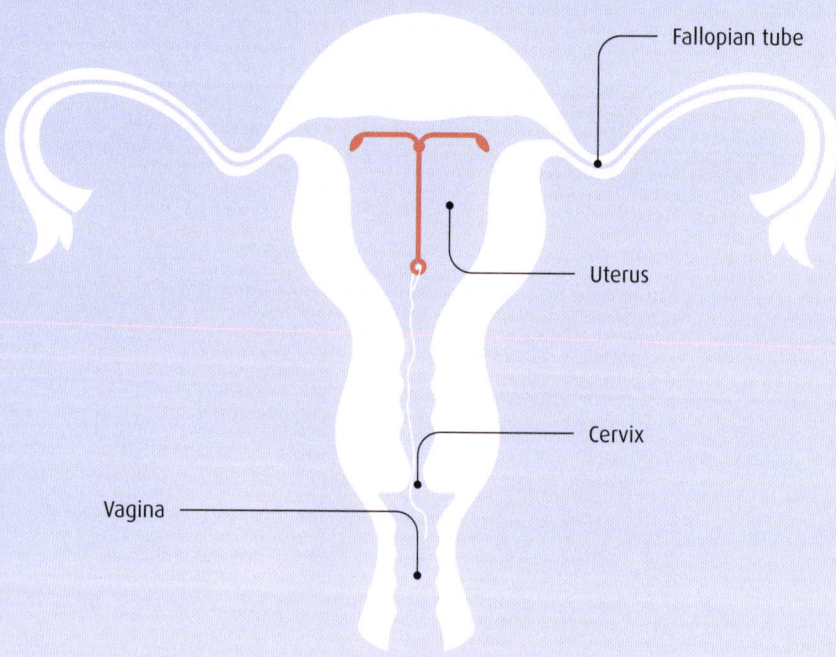

Copper IUDs

Since IUDs do not disrupt ovulation or your hormonal balance, vaginal secretions (cervical mucus and vaginal discharge) are still present throughout your cycle. However, with periods often being heavier and longer, the prolonged presence of blood (pH 7.4) changes the natural acidity of the vagina (pH 4); the flora can suffer, leading to a greater risk of vaginosis.

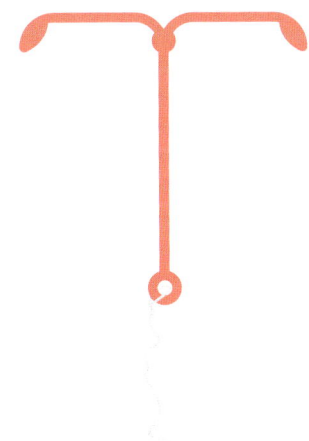

Progesterone IUDs

IUDs vary depending on the hormone dosage. The main ones include Kyleena, which has a low dosage, and Mirena, which has a higher dosage. IUDs operate on two levels: 1) the cervical mucus thickens, making it impermeable to the passage of sperm; 2) the endometrium (the tissue that lines the inside of the uterus) becomes unfit for implantation. This double "lock" gives progesterone IUDs greater efficiency compared to their cooper counterparts. Kyleena does not interfere with ovulation; the amount of hormones that passes through the blood during a month is equivalent to the amount that would transfer from a mini-dose pill tablet if you were to leave it under your tongue for the same period of time. In contrast, Mirena, which does not block the menstrual cycle, can nevertheless interfere with ovulation. Under the effect of progesterone, cervical mucus thickens, which occurs naturally after ovulation. Gone is the slimy and transparent discharge — you will only find the cloudy and sticky kind!

Opposite to what happens with copper IUDs, periods disappear for 9 out of 10 women. With Kyleena, their flow decreases significantly until it is minimal or non-existent. Progesterone continuously diffused in the endometrium makes it very thin, which explains why there is only a small amount of bleeding.

Condoms

Female or male, condoms are made of latex or polyurethane. If you are allergic to latex, you will find out soon enough because your vagina and vulva will quickly swell, and you will feel an intense burning sensation. In that case, there is only one option: Switch to polyurethane condoms. Whichever you use, for the sake of your vaginal mucosa, choose lubricated condoms.

Remember that condoms are the only means for preventing sexually transmitted infections, but as contraception, they are not always enough within the normal conditions of use. For a condom to be effective birth control, it must meet several conditions: Use a condom no matter what day of the cycle you're on (there are no days without risk), choose the right size, put it on correctly at the start of sex, remove it immediately after ejaculation (before the erection starts to shrink), and check that it remained intact and the sperm has not leaked. If there's the slightest doubt, use an emergency contraceptive, like the morning-after pill (such as Plan B One-Step or Next Choice) or have a copper IUD inserted in the five days following sex.

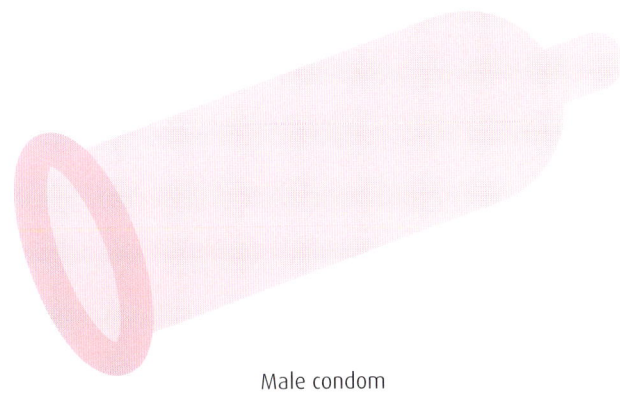

Male condom

Use of female condoms is not widespread, but if you decide to use this method, being familiar with your vagina will serve you particularly well when inserting the small ring to the very back of your vagina and then applying the condom against the walls of your vagina with a finger. Female condoms are single use. If possible, put one in a few hours before sex, which will help it adhere to the vaginal walls (so much for spontaneity!), and guide your partner's penis so that, in the heat of the moment, it enters into the condom and not between it and the vaginal wall. After sex, remove the condom by twisting the end of the ring while avoiding all leaks of sperm. It's almost as complicated as putting together a piece of furniture from a certain Swedish brand, wouldn't you say?

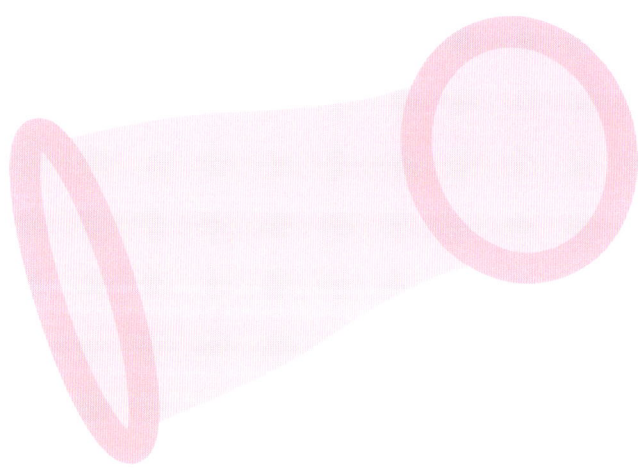

Female condom

Placement of a Female Condom

1 Pinch the middle of the ring between your thumb and index finger to form a figure-eight shape and insert it into the vagina.

2 The opening must stay outside of the vagina and properly cover the labia area.

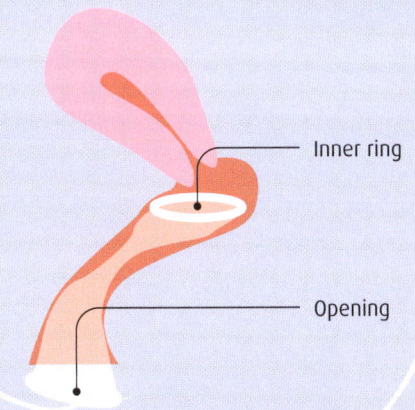

Diaphragms and Spermicides

Diaphragms look similar to menstrual cups. They have a small silicone cup that you fit over the cervix before sex. Alone, they are not 100 percent effective in preventing sperm from getting through, which is why it is recommended to always use a spermicide with a diaphragm. Like the female condom, a diaphragm requires that you know your body well enough to properly place it over the cervix. To do so, you must choose the correct size; in general, small for those who have not given birth, and medium or large for those who have. If you're unsure about your size, ask your gynecologist.

Diaphragms and spermicides are "light" contraceptives meant for times of low fertility.

Note that diaphragms do not protect against sexually transmitted infections.

Spermicides are products that you put inside the vagina immediately before sex. They come in the following forms: ovules, vaginal creams, single-dose applicators and sponges. Spermicides work by neutralizing sperm, but they are not 100 percent effective. They are like a "light' form of contraception, reserved for times when risk of pregnancy is low. During the period after childbirth, for example, fertility is low until the first ovulation, which occurs 15 days before the first period returns — and is completely unpredictable! In perimenopause, fertility is also low — but not zero, so be careful. During these times, when the vagina is sometimes a bit dry, spermicides provide extra lubrication. However, an intolerance to chloride or benzalkonium, which are found in spermicides, is possible.

The Vagina and Contraceptives | 79

Diaphragm

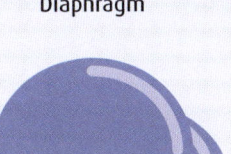

Spermicides

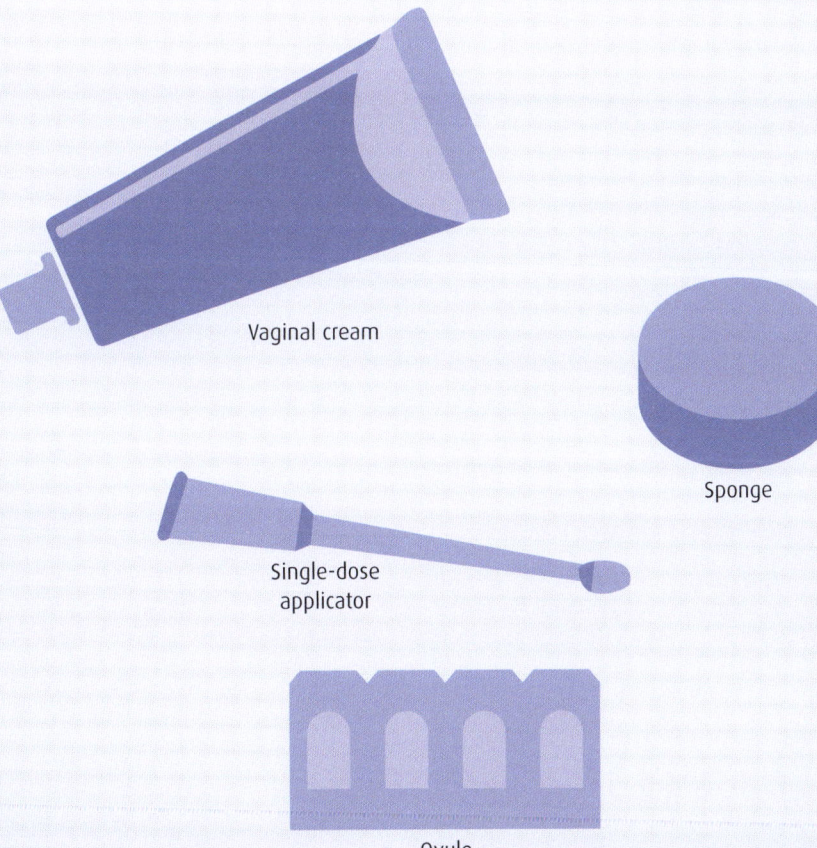

Vaginal cream

Sponge

Single-dose applicator

Ovule

Placement of a Diaphragm

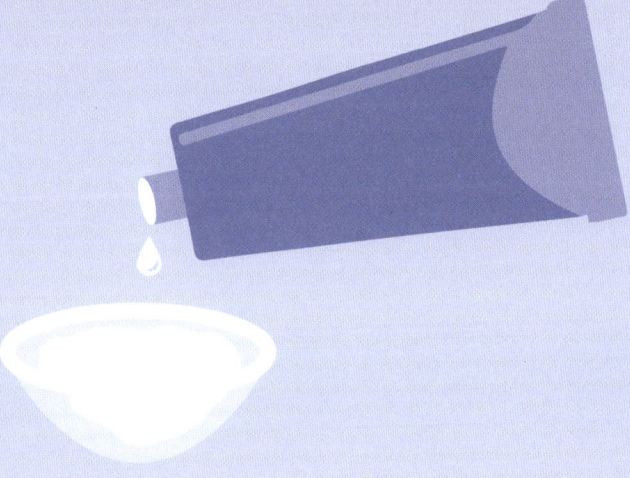

Add spermicide

Pinch the diaphragm

The Vagina and Contraceptives | 81

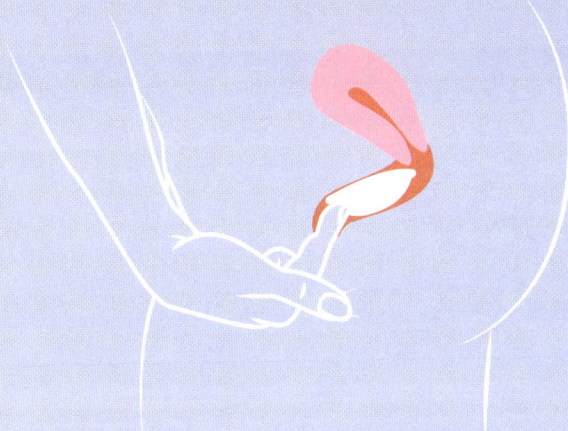

Push the diaphragm upward.

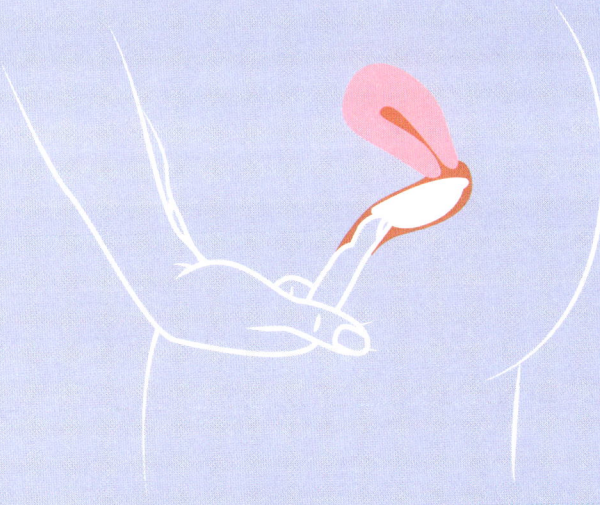

It's in!

Vaginal Problems
▌Vaginismus ▌

Many conditions can affect the vagina, and that impact can go beyond the physical. Such conditions can also affect the intimate relationship between the woman and her body as well as the relationship between sexual partners.

Too often, vaginismus is not discussed because the women who are affected feel shame and guilt and don't dare talk about it. However, this is a common sexual disorder, affecting 1 in 200 couples and 1 in 20 couples seeking medical intervention for infertility. The numbers are, in fact, higher in Muslim countries, as shown in a 2008 Turkish study that reports 1 percent to 10 percent of young couples suffer from it.

Vaginismus is characterized by a spasm of the pelvic floor muscles, preventing all penetration — not a finger, tampon, or speculum, and certainly not a penis. This fear of penetration is triggered by a simple touch, which contracts the perineal muscles via a strong muscle spasm. The most common form of vaginismus is called primary vaginismus (which is inherent, meaning it has always existed no matter the circumstance or the partner); there is no cause for this phobia. In contrast, secondary vaginismus occurs in women who were previously able to have sex with full penetration; in that case, it is recommended to seek out the traumatic causal event. A woman affected by vaginismus, even with all the will in the world, will not be able to relax her perineal muscles.

Fear distorts all sensations — whereas a woman unaffected by vaginismus will simply feel a stretch, a woman suffering from vaginismus will feel unbearable pain.

However, contrary to what you may think, vaginismus is not an exclusively female sexual or gynecological problem — it concerns both people in a couple. To illustrate my point, I share with you a definition given to me by a Genevan midwife I met many years ago: Vaginismus is the story of a visitor who would like to come in but doesn't dare, and a host who wants to entertain but can't. In other words, it takes two to tango!

Don't think, however, that this couple doesn't have a sex life; desire (even if it ends abruptly) and pleasure are part of the interaction — only penetration is sorely missing from the equation. Different kinds of sex can be introduced to satisfy the woman but will nevertheless leave the man unfulfilled.

It's often a childhood desire to "be like everyone else" that pushes a woman to get help. Although every woman and man have their own unique experience, let me tell you, in a somewhat exaggerated way, what I was able to observe from the rehabilitation of more than 100 couples that I've followed

> **Vaginismus is an uncontrollable spasm of the perineal muscles.**

during my career. The typical consultation that I will describe helps provide an overall picture of both parties' attitudes and explains how vaginismus shapes their relationship. If you suffer from vaginismus, you will probably be able to relate with the following.

I invite you into the privacy of a consultation...

Most often, a woman comes for consultation not with her husband but with her shame and guilt about their marriage not being "consummated," as they say. Or a woman seeks out a consultation pushed by her desire to get pregnant, but with a heavy heart and convinced she is alone in this and that she's a failure.

She sits upright, on the edge of her seat, legs crossed. Behind an obvious shyness that reveals further embarrassment, I often find a strong, determined woman. She has never used a tampon and even less explored herself intimately. She is not usually frigid; she has experienced clitoral orgasms, and her desire, although hampered, is intact.

Her husband is gentle, patient, respectful and understanding. Like his young, virgin wife, this lover does not have much sexual experience either. He feels helpless, not knowing what to do, especially since sometimes both were raised in a traditional culture, valuing virginity before marriage. But they remained optimistic — for a long time, a very long time, too long of a time — because our tortured couple thought that with time everything would work out. Alas, vaginismus is persistent and is justly defined by its longevity! The couple revolves around vaginismus and it defines their entire marital relationship. By contrast, if a couple in which the husband lacks experience and the wife has an intense fear of having sex for the first time seek out a consultation in the first few months of their marriage, vaginismus will likely be only a bad memory.

So yes, those with vaginismus can be successfully rehabilitated by trained professionals: gynecologists, midwives, physiotherapists

> **Vaginismus is a sexual disorder that affects the couple, not just the woman.**

and sexologists. Rehabilitation is always a mind-body process — this means using touch when necessary, but never with force, in a very gradual way and with a great deal of will. Each therapist applies their own techniques, which often involve relaxation, body awareness (with a focus on exploring your vagina), perineal therapy and use of vaginal dilators. Surgery is never, and I mean never, the solution. Hymenotomy (surgical opening of the hymen) is for hymen deformities. Vaginismus could be interpreted as the last stage of dyspareunia, the medical term for pain during sexual intercourse.

Pain During Sex

What woman hasn't experienced, even for a moment, pain during sex? The vagina itself is not sensitive, but everything around it is — thus, a certain number of unpleasant sensations are attributed to the vagina.

To make things simple, dyspareunia (pain during sex) can be split into two categories: pain felt at the vaginal opening during penetration (superficial dyspareunia) or pain felt deep inside (deep dyspareunia).

> **It's important to distinguish between deep and superficial dyspareunia.**

Deep Pain

If the pain comes and goes, try to note if it is happening at certain times of your cycle. During ovulation, the ovary that releases the follicle or the small amount of post-ovulation discharge can be the cause of pain. If the pain happens only during certain positions, it could be caused by the impact of the penis against the particularly sensitive zone of the posterior fornix that faces the isthmus of a retroverted uterus. The uterine isthmus is the passageway between the cervix and the uterine body, and it has a ton of nerves. When the uterus is tilted toward the back, the isthmus lies exactly in the trajectory of the penis — which would explain the pain! If the pain, whether dull or sharp, occurs during all sexual encounters, and especially if it persists outside of sex, a gynecological visit is required, as it may be an organic disease, such as endometriosis or a pelvic infection.

Retroverted Uterus

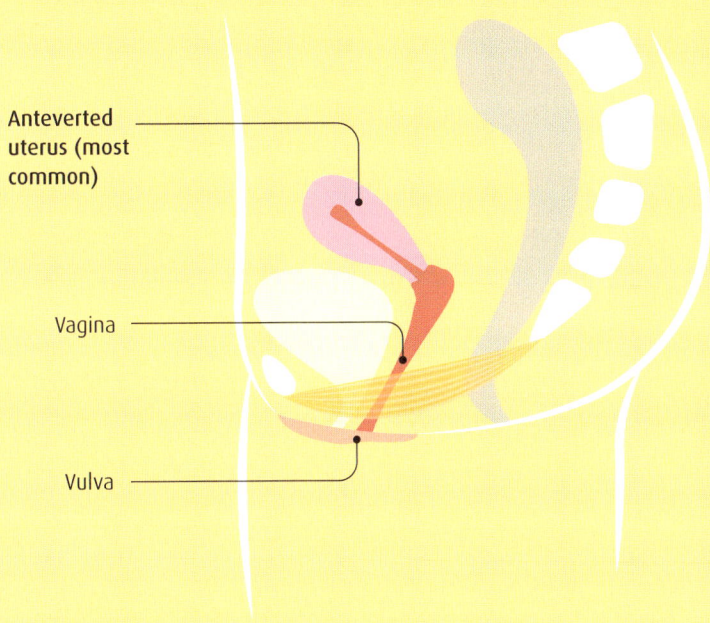

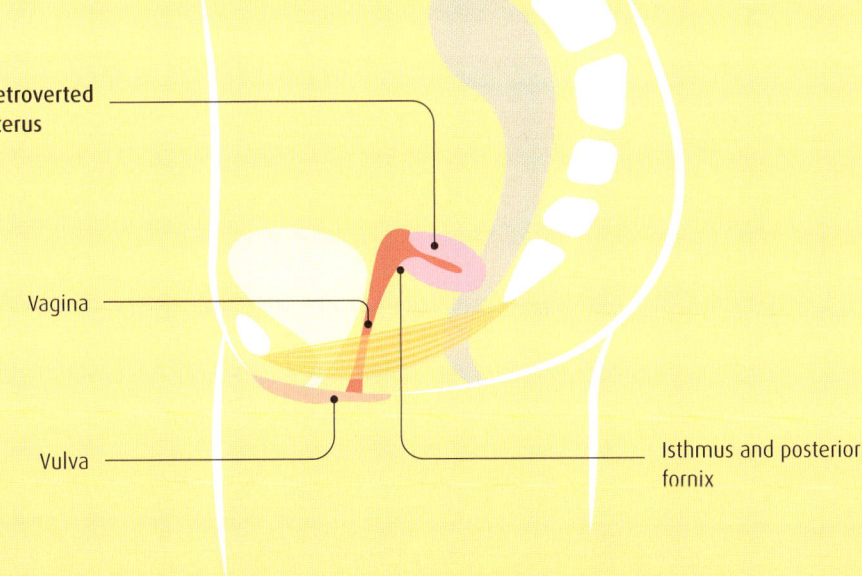

Endometriosis, a common disorder that affects 1 in 10 women of reproductive age, occurs when endometrium (the tissue that lines the inside of the uterus) grows outside of the uterus. These growths act like the endometrium and bleed during a period, causing pain.

They can cause adenomyosis in the uterine muscle, which leads to aggravated dysmenorrhea, meaning periods that become more painful from one cycle to the next. These clusters of endometrial cells can form cysts on the ovaries, called endometriomas, and they can can cause infertility or an ectopic pregnancy in the fallopian tube they obstruct. They can also end up throughout the pelvis, bladder, digestive tract just below the liver and even in the skin, forming bluish nodules. In the intestines, endometriosis causes pain, which is typically stronger in the second phase of the cycle and during a period but tends to become chronic over time. When endometriosis affects the tissue around the uterus and vagina, it can cause deep pain during sex. Endometriosis is a disorder of varying severity among women and is underdiagnosed.

Pelvic inflammatory disease, on the other hand, causes abnormal vaginal discharge (sometimes with pus), constant pelvic pain that is exacerbated during sex and, in certain cases, a fever.

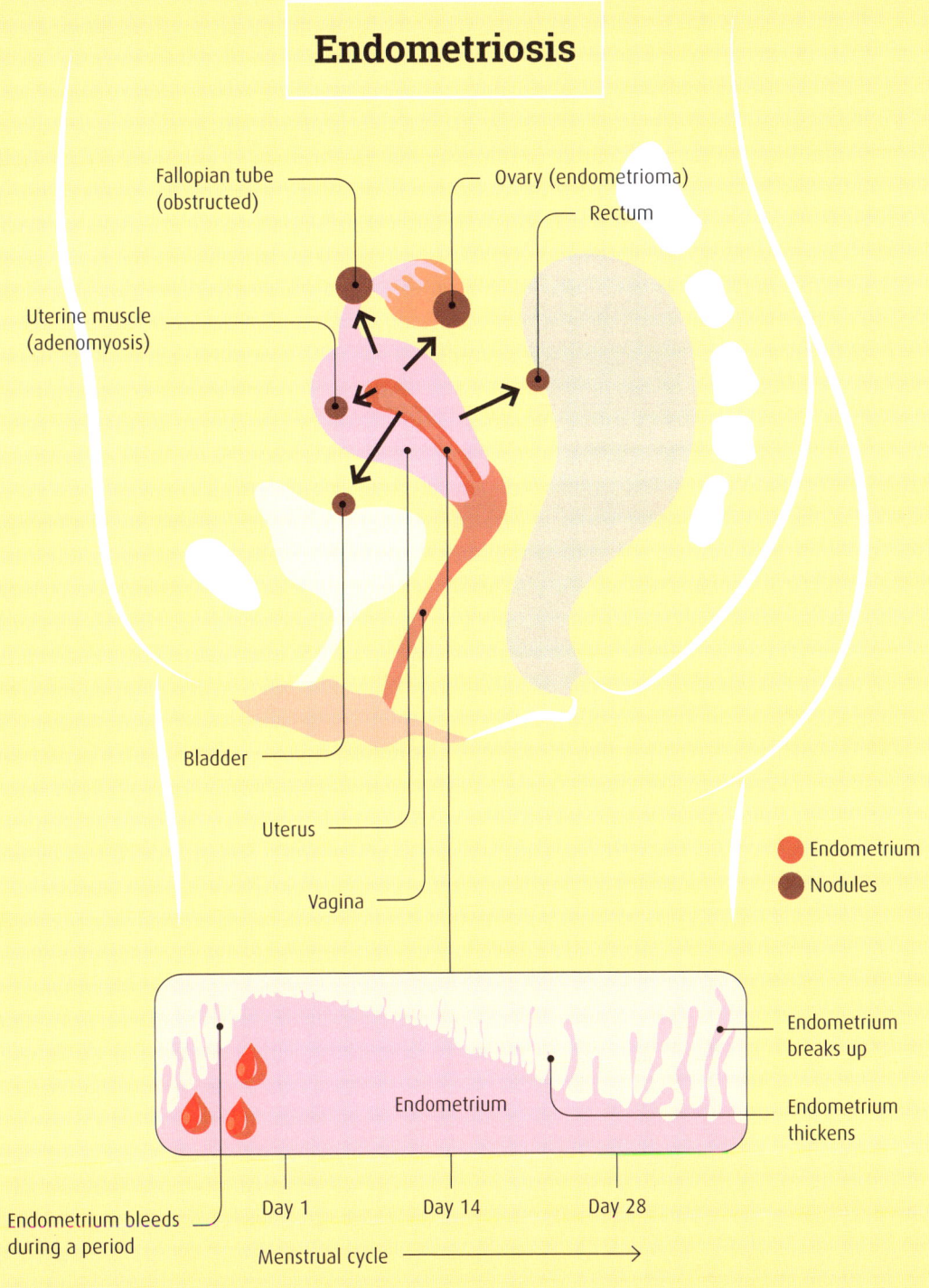

Superficial Pain

Women do not always feel pain in the vagina. The vulva and vestibule can also be painful areas. All it takes is vulvovaginitis — the most common type is mycosis (a yeast infection) — for sex to burn! Almost all women are familiar with that happening, but have you ever heard of lichen sclerosus or vestibulitis?

Lichen Sclerosus

Lichen sclerosus (LS) is a dermatological condition of the vulva. Since it affects mostly menopausal women, younger women who complain about pain during penetration are not diagnosed early. The cause of lichen sclerosus is still a mystery — it is thought to be caused by an immune imbalance — but it is certain that this disorder is not infectious, and there's no risk of spread. In short, you could say that it's a chronic disorder that can be treated but not cured. In addition to dyspareunia, LS manifests in chronic pruritus (itching) accompanied by an anatomical change of the vulva. The labia minora shrink until, at an advanced stage, they disappear entirely. The mucus of the vestibule turns pearly white and cracks easily. After a thorough examination, a gynecologist or dermatologist will be able to make a diagnosis. A local treatment of cortisone, for life, stabilizes the disorder and restores vulvar comfort. Very rare vulvar cancers always begin with lichen, but corticoid treatments are enough to prevent this complication.

> **Lichen sclerosus is a chronic dermatological condition.**

Vestibulitis

Vestibulitis, which mostly affects younger women, causes localized vestibule pain, which is exacerbated during sex and sometimes reignited by walking or moving. Pudendal neuralgia, much rarer than vestibulitis, has similar symptoms. However, a light touch with the help of a cotton swab on the sensitive area that results in pain is specific to vestibulitis. This cotton swab test is done in a gynecologist's office, but it can also be done at home. Just position one end of the stick on the area (often the lower part of the vestibule) to determine if there is sharp pain. Of course, you must follow-up with a medical consultation, but this will help you start to put a name to your pain.

Even though we do not know the cause of this mysterious and all too often overlooked disorder, there are effective treatments. Your gynecologist can prescribe a vitamin E based protective cream, for example, to apply to the vestibule, which will bring some relief. Perineal rehabilitation sessions with a trained physiotherapist or midwife are equally very helpful. As with vaginismus, psychological counseling is necessary because this condition is chronic — even if it eventually disappears after several months or years — and, above all, because it has an impact on your sexual and emotional life.

> **Vestibulitis treatment is multifaceted and includes gynecology, perineal rehabilitation training and psychological counseling.**

> **Vaginal Dryness**
>
> We have already discussed vaginal dryness, which happens for many reasons. Let's review what we learned with the help of a little quiz.

1 **Why is vaginal mucosa dry or very dry?**

Due to a lack of estrogen, a lack of stimulation or a change in vaginal flora.

2 **Why is lubrication a challenge during sex?**

It depends on arousal, the state of the vagina and a domino effect.

3 **The domino effect — what's that all about?**

It's a vicious circle that comes about when there is insufficient lubrication: the vagina and surrounding area is dry, so it hurts, and that hurdle disrupts the arousal process. Lubrication, which is proportional to how aroused you are, will decrease, pleasure will drop during sex, interest in continuing will wane, the number of sexual encounters will decrease, which will weaken the vaginal mucosa even more, which will become dryer, and so on.

The Domino Effect

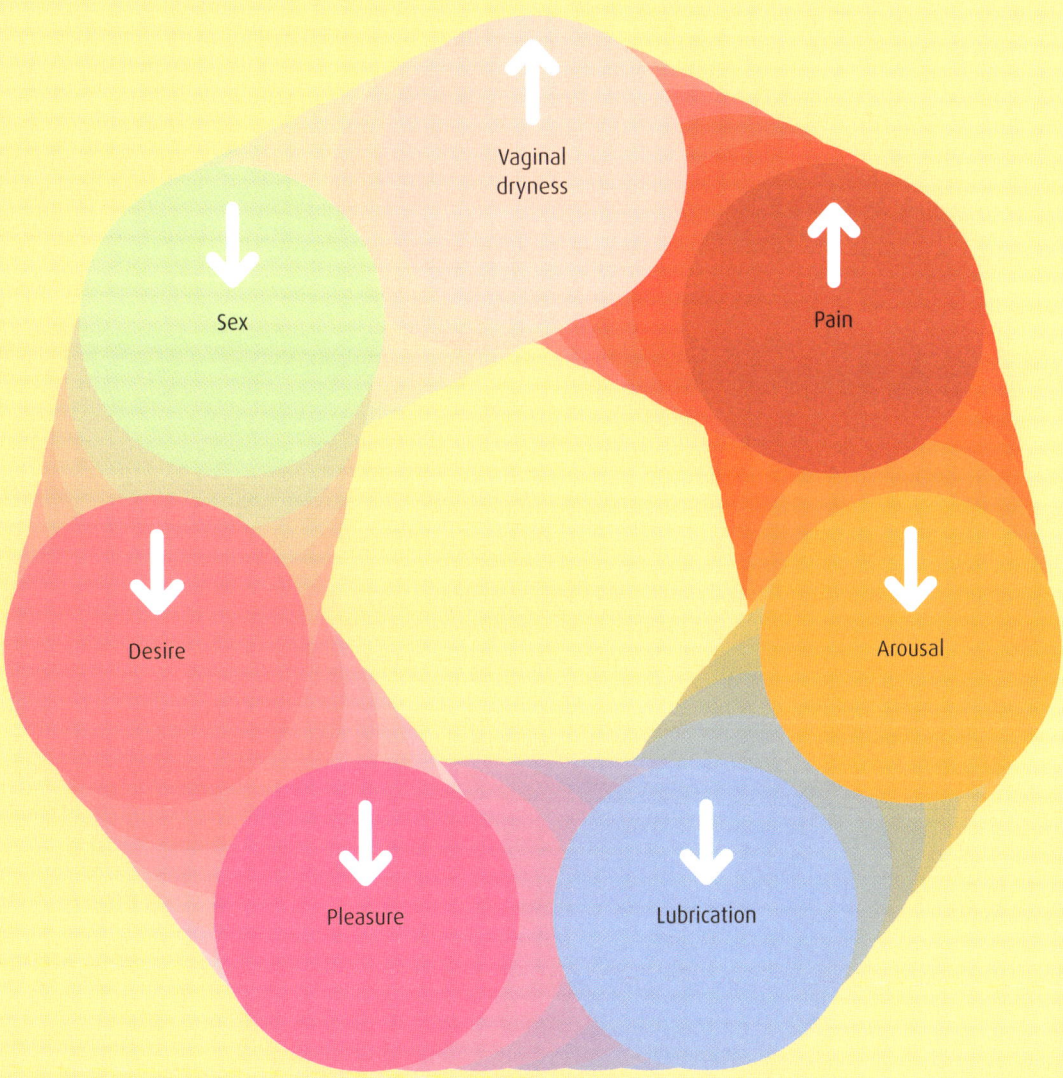

Does vaginal dryness impact day-to-day life?
Yes, and even more than you can understand. A study conducted in six European countries aiming to evaluate menopause symptoms showed that vaginal dryness has a negative impact on sex in 20 percent of couples, affects self-esteem for 50 percent of women and results in a decrease in sex drive that is characterized by low morale, no desire to engage and a diminished zest for life.[3]

 Okay, now what?
Adapt! Extend foreplay, use lube to get things revving and keep your partner in mind.

 How can I avoid vaginal dryness?
Add some of the following options to your shopping list:
• A product that is appropriate for feminine hygiene.
• A protective cream or organic St. John's Wort or calendula essential oil. However, never apply essential oil directly to mucus or inside the vagina without diluting beforehand in a base oil.
• A hydrophilic or hyaluronic acid-based moisturizing vaginal gel (such as Replens).
• Organic aloe vera gel.

 And if that isn't enough?
Make an appointment. Your gynecologist may recommend hyaluronic acid injections or endovaginal laser treatment. And remember to have regular sex!

3. L. Nappi, "Women's Perception of Sexuality Around the Menopause: Outcomes of a European Telephone Survey," *European Journal of Obstetrics & Gynecology and Reproductive Biology* 137 (2008): 10–16.

Prolapse

The word "prolapse" is a medical term for what is more commonly referred to as a hernia.

There are three types of prolapse: cystocele, when the bladder shifts from its natural position and partially or fully descends into the vagina (anterior wall); rectocele, which involves the rectum (posterior wall); and, more rarely, hysterocele, when the whole uterus drops down.

The vagina is particularly exposed, with its walls connected to the bladder and rectum walls. When the elasticity of these tissues deteriorates, the walls cave in and protrude outward — at first, only when pushing (stage 1) and then permanently (stage 3).

Even rarer, the cervix protrudes from the vagina, either because it is too long or because the entire uterus has taken the elevator to the ground floor.

Prolapse is a medical term referring to the descent of an organ.

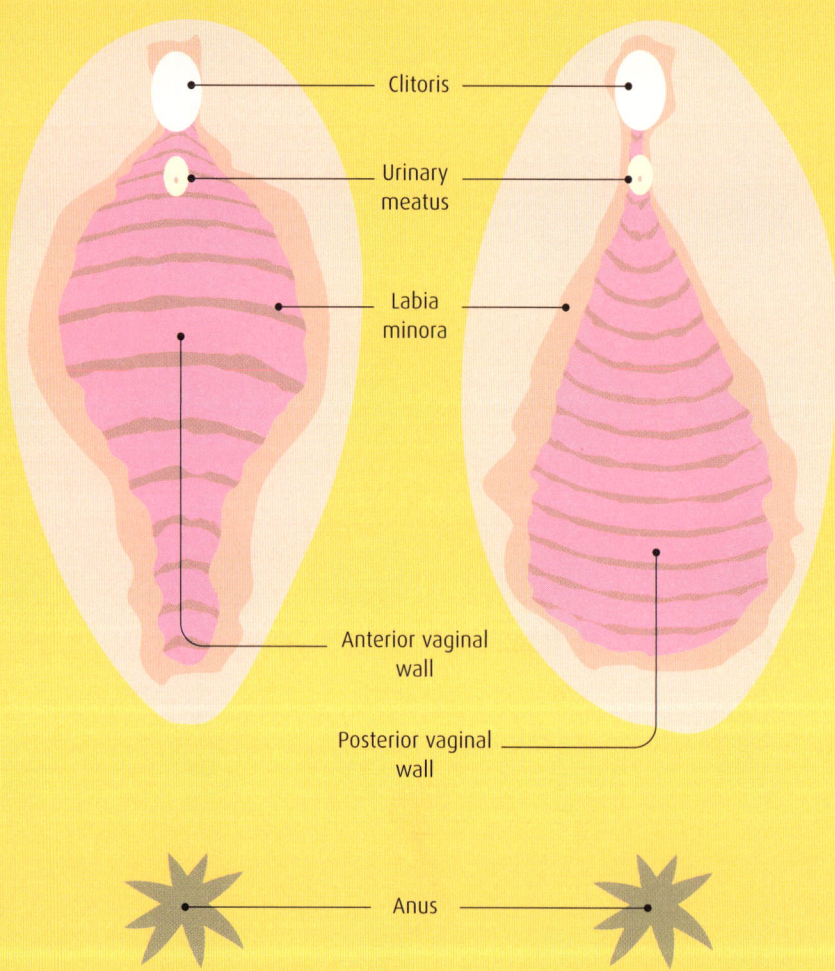

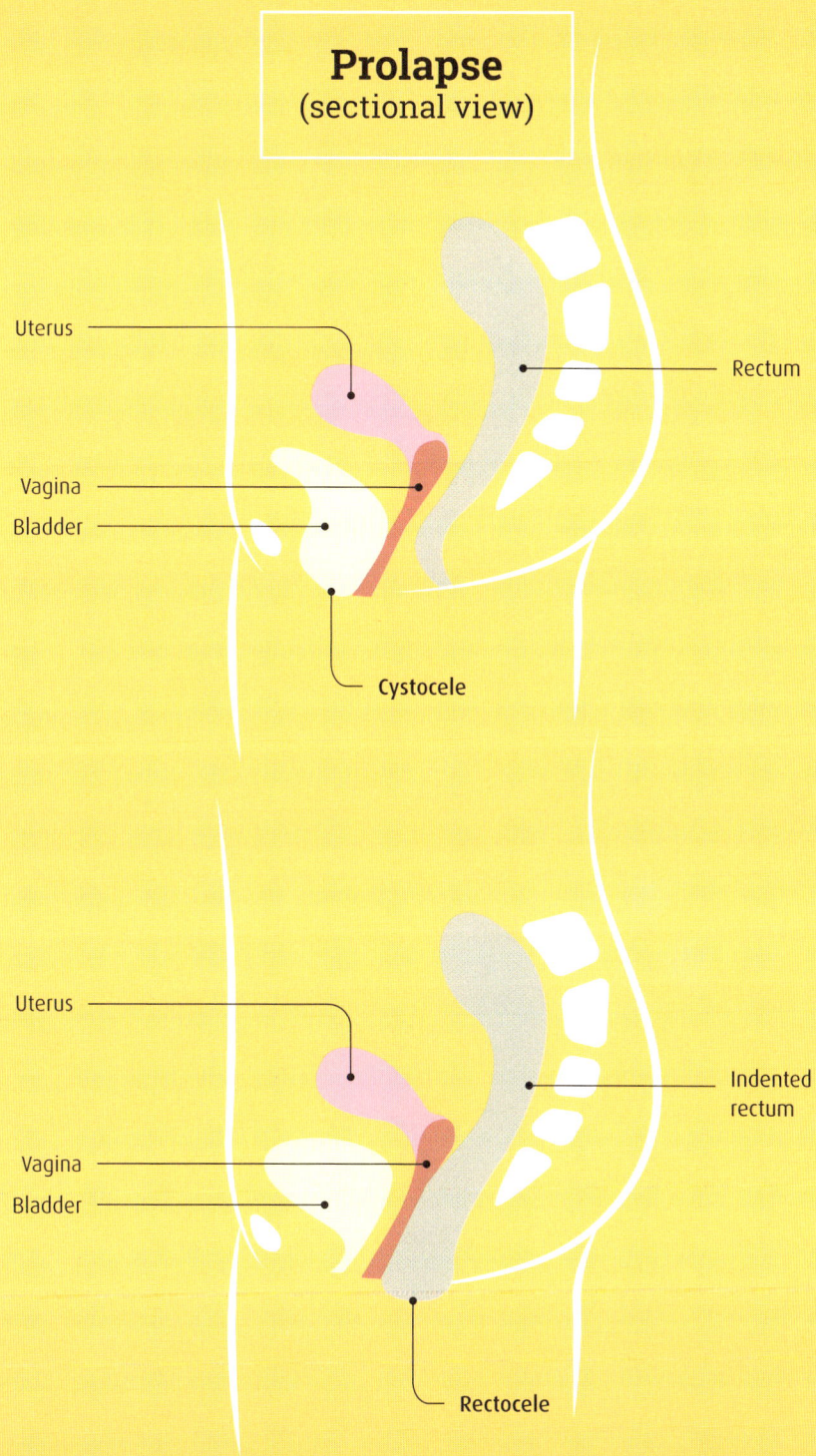

How Do You Avoid a "Fall"?

With prevention, by avoiding as much as possible anything that can push organs and the vagina downward: obesity, big babies (in the case of gestational diabetes), chronic constipation, heavy lifting, improper physical activity or playing sports without abdominal or perineal support. To bulk up your abdominals, start by engaging your perineal muscles, and then do your exercises while exhaling. Perineal rehabilitation, even if it doesn't return the vagina to its original elasticity or pull the bladder back up into the pelvis, has great merit. It strengthens the perineal muscles to maintain this little world inside — that's already a big deal, wouldn't you say?

Perineal Rehabilitation

There are three methods: a manual method and two using vaginal probes. The manual method is done at a midwife's or physiotherapist's office. There is much to be said for including hypopressive exercises, which teach one how to reduce the abdominal pressure that tends to push organs downward.[4]

Functional Electrical Stimulation (FES) involves electrically stimulating the perineal muscles with a vaginal probe. Don't worry, there's no electrical shock!

Finally, biofeedback allows you to feel, contract and control the muscles, to interpret their contraction and to evaluate their progress. It is possible to practice these rehabilitation methods either a with a professional or at home. The latest devices on the market connect to practical and easy-to-use apps. The devices have proven effectiveness, and, because there is more engagement, the risk of stopping sessions prematurely also decreases.

Perineal rehabilitation can take place at a midwife's or physiotherapist's office.

---

[4] The referenced specialist on this subject is Dr. Bernadette de Gasquet.

Surgery

Prolapse surgery is recommended when the descent of your organ is bothering you to the point where you feel something rubbing against your underwear. In the case of rectocele or cystocele without incontinence, surgery only involves the vagina. A diamond-shape piece is excised from the wall, and the sides are stitched back up, the excess tissue having been removed. After the surgery, you should refrain from heavy lifting and you must wait one month before having sex. You should not feel any pain because intravaginal scars are not very sensitive.

Urinary problems are not typically linked to cystocele, but urinary incontinence, particularly stress urinary incontinence, is fairly common. In that case, after having precisely identified the type of incontinence by urodynamic testing (a specialized bladder test), the placement of a sling that lifts the bladder and corrects urinary incontinence will be recommended. The intervention involves threading a strip of mesh, approximately ½ inch (1.5 cm) wide, under the urethra to lift it up into the pelvis. And voilà, your bladder is well placed once again! For this technique, only three small incisions are necessary, one vaginal and two in the inguinal crease or behind the pubis. This operation, under general anesthesia, is an outpatient procedure.

> **Surgery is recommended only if you experience daily discomfort.**

Sparc® sling

Prolapse Surgery

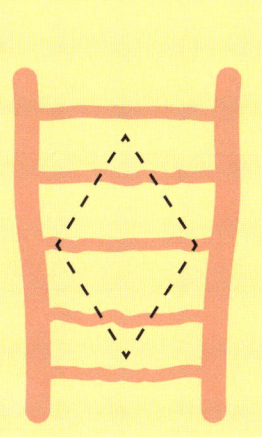
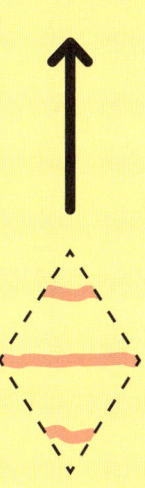
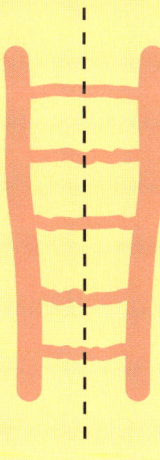

Cervical Diseases

Thanks to Pap smears, cervical cancer has become rare, but there are still many cases of cervical dysplasia.

Dysplasia is a risk factor for cervical cancer and should be treated. Oftentimes, simple monitoring is enough, and recovery takes 12 to 18 months.

> **Conization barely changes the anatomy of the cervix.**

If it doesn't heal, the lesion will be surgically removed, in most cases under local anesthesia, by conization. This procedure is done with the help of a diathermic snare, which simultaneously cuts and cauterizes a small cone from the cervix, removing the diseased part. The cervix mends immediately; it's just a little bit smaller. Post-operative care is usually minimal, with a small risk of bleeding around the eighth day that you'll need to watch out for. The more tissue that's spared in the procedure, the less consequences there will be for fertility, childbirth and pregnancy. When it comes to sex, there will be no change in sensation.

Conization

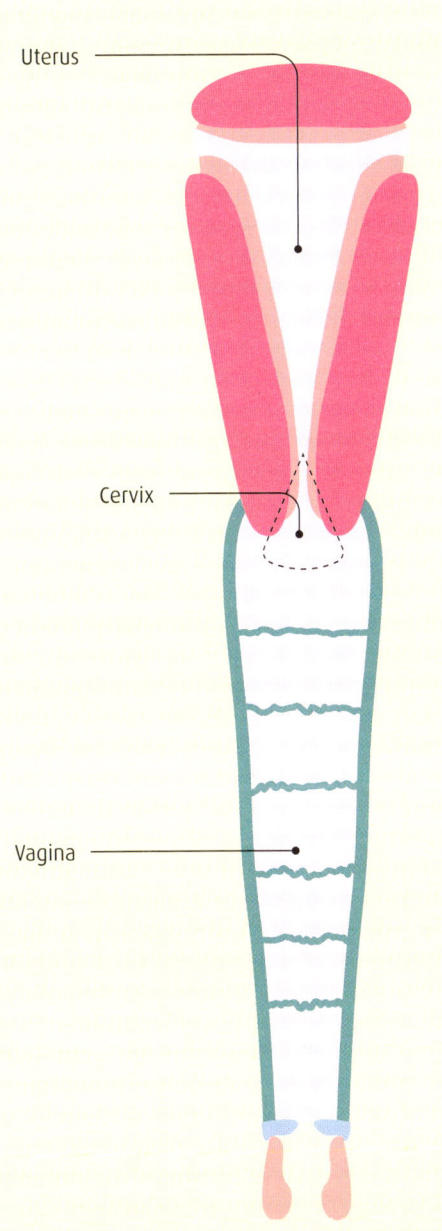
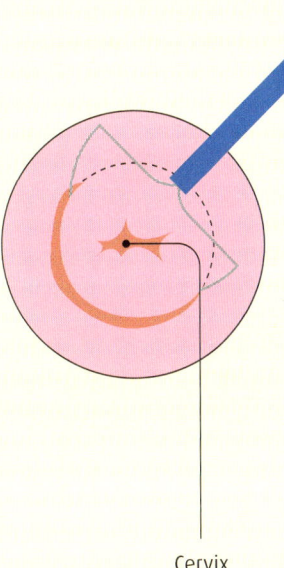

■ Uterine Diseases ■

Fibroids, cancers and bleeding sometimes necessitate the sacrifice of the uterus: a hysterectomy.

There are vaginal hysterectomies and abdominal hysterectomies. If the condition is not cancerous and the uterus is not too large, a vaginal hysterectomy is performed, in which case post-operative care is simpler. The choice to remove the ovaries or not at the same time is decided on a case-by-case basis.

What happens to the vagina after a hysterectomy? For a sub-total hysterectomy, the surgeon will leave the cervix, which will not alter the vagina anatomically. However, regular screening for cervical cancer (Pap test) is required. For a total hysterectomy, the cervix is also removed. Deep in the vagina, a straight-lined scar can be felt in place of the cervix. When it comes to sex, nothing will change — neither your sensations nor your moves!

Hysterectomy

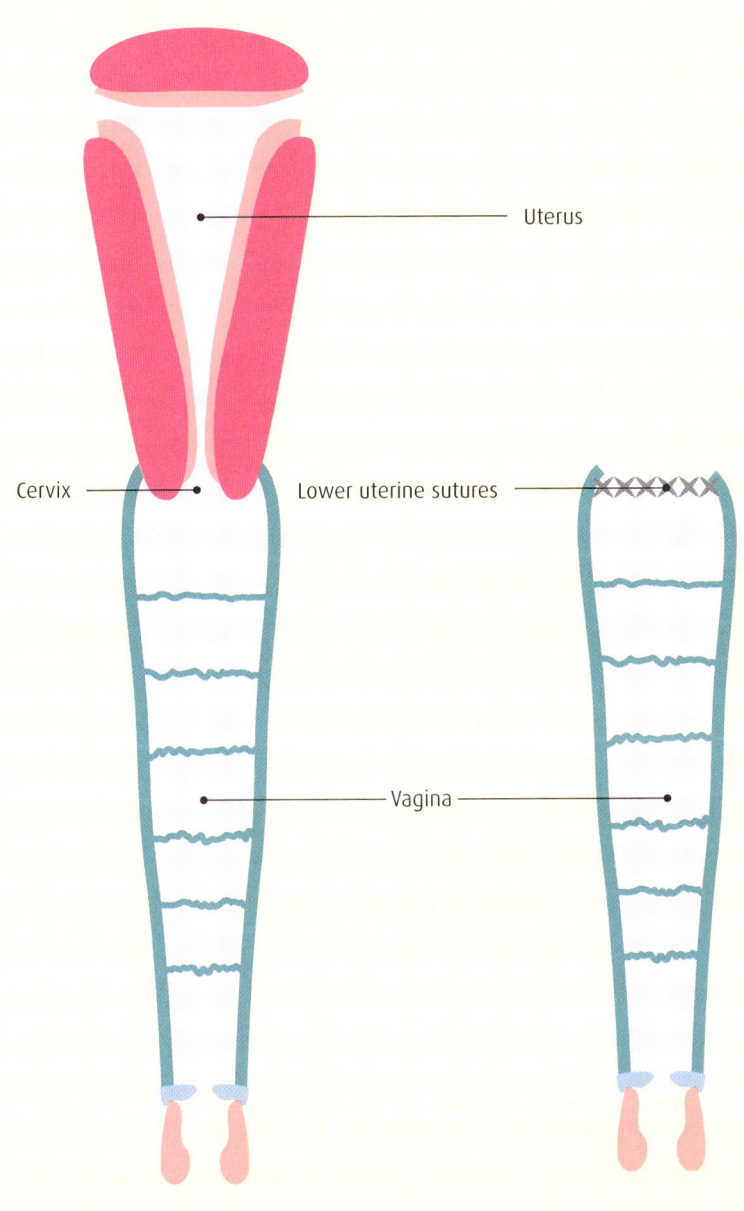

Vulvovaginitis

When it stings, burns, leaks or smells awful, you have only one thought: kick down the door to your gynecologist's office for relief as soon as possible!

The guilty party, the one that prevents you from sleeping because of a furious urge to scratch or that fills your underwear with an unpleasant deposit — that's vulvovaginitis. It's an infection of the vagina and vulva caused by an imbalance in the vaginal flora, but it is not a sexually transmitted infection (STI). Given that vulvovaginitis is most often caused by a fungus (mycosis), many women refer to anything that causes leaks, itching or abnormal bacteria growth as a yeast infection. If you have these symptoms, you will be highly tempted to find relief with the first antifungal ovules that you come across on the pharmacy shelves. Big mistake! There is nothing like retuning to the vicious circle that is vulvovaginitis that keeps coming back. Therefore, it is particularly important to know how to recognize the different kinds of vulvovaginitis, their cause, their treatment and, while we're at it, how to prevent it from coming back. Such an infection, at least temporarily, will impact your sex life. The problem becomes critical when the infection keeps returning — and the time between two vulvovaginitis flare-ups decreases and the time between sexual encounters increases. In that case, comprehensive, psychosomatic and even serological care is necessary.

> **Not all types of vulvovaginitis are mycoses!**

Mycosis

This vulvovaginal infection is caused by an overgrowth of a yeast (or fungus, if you prefer to more bucolic term) called Candida albicans, which can be found all over the body (the intestines, the mouth and, of course, the vagina). It's mere presence together with Döderlein's bacilli is not by itself enough to cause mycosis (more commonly known as a yeast infection), but if they settle in and get comfortable, and show up along with a burning sensation and discharge that resembles curdled milk on a scarlet-red vestibule — that's another story!

As you now know, you cannot "catch" yeast infections; they develop on their own. The depletion of lactobacilli allows *Candida albicans* to completely take over the vaginal flora, which can occur for the following reasons: use of antibiotics, extensive time spent in a pool, change in diet, lowered immune system, lack of estrogen due to menopause or birth control, or simply partially treated acute mycosis. If the symptoms are happening outside of the body, in the vulva, it means the infection also affects the vaginal mucosa, which, when examined with a speculum, will be covered in a curdled-looking white discharge (resembling cottage cheese). An antifungal cream can relieve the burning sensation, but it will not cure mycosis. For that reason, it is imperative to always choose the correct vaginal ovule. You will generally be prescribed an ovule along with a cream to apply for one week and your doctor may recommend a feminine hygiene wash with a basic pH balance — because Candida has a nasty tendency to flare up under treatment, releasing an acidic substance called candidin. So don't be surprised if in the hours after starting treatment you notice a brief worsening of symptoms. Rest assured, it's only temporary.

If you develop only one yeast infection per year or less, and the previous description applies to you, you can ask your pharmacist directly for a comprehensive antifungal treatment (cream and ovule). If you are unsure or it is a recurring problem, make an appointment with your health care provider. Your doctor may take a sample of the bacteria from your vagina to identify the bacteria responsible for your vulvovaginitis and prescribe the appropriate treatment for you. If you have four or more yeast infections per year, it's recurrent mycosis. To manage it, first the vaginal flora needs to be rebalanced with either locally or systemically administered probiotics (rich in lactobacilli). Afterward, a preventative antifungal treatment is recommended, to be administered orally or vaginally once a month, for example. In complementary medicine, I fully recommend the following homeopathic treatment: three Monilia Albicans 9 CH tablets a day for three months.

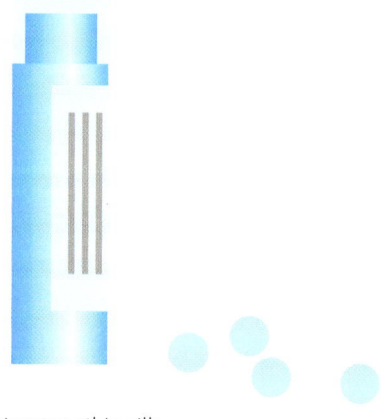

Homeopathic pills

Vaginosis

Second on the list of vulvovaginitis offenders is vaginosis. This typical imbalance of vaginal flora, linked to the increase of pH, encourages the growth of certain native bacteria, of which the most common is *Gardnerella vaginalis*. Symptoms include an abundance of abnormally colored, slightly irritating and liquid discharge, whose distinguishing characteristic is its bad odor, like that of rotten fish.

The factors promoting vaginosis include the presence of blood in the vagina (spotting, heavy periods or frequent periods), a copper IUD, frequent sex or vaginal douching (the latter should be done away with in all cases!).

Treatment requires imidazole antibiotics, either taken for one week (Flagyl) or as your doctor recommends. Your prescription may leave you feeling sick to your stomach, but you'll feel much better soon. The pills may be accompanied by Flagyl ovules. The vagina's natural pH balance will be restored thanks to tablets or vaginal gels with acidic pH.

There is only one situation where the odor is more unbearable than with vaginosis: the forgotten tampon. Patients always say the same thing: "Doctor, I wash myself 10 times a day and it still smells so bad!" That's enough to make a diagnosis and go fishing for the tampon — holding one's breath if possible.

It can sometimes be difficult to distinguish between a vaginosis that is accompanied by slight burning and only a mild odor and a light micosis that is accompanied by a slightly unusual odor. A test kit, based on the color the stick turns, can help you determine between the two infections. It's a practical method because, in the case of a first vaginosis, you can improve the situation simply by applying an over-the-counter gel or tablet based on the recommendation of your doctor or pharmacist.

The "Outsiders"

Besides mycosis and vaginosis, there are some (non-specific) vaginal infections that, like these first two, are the result of an imbalance of flora cause by naturally occurring bacteria in the vagina. We're talking about vulvovaginitis caused by *Escherichia coli* and streptococcus.

For vaginal infections, it's all a matter of balancing the different bacteria!

You may have heard of *Escherichia coli*, also called colibacillus and shortened to E. coli, in reference to urinary infections. It can also cause abnormally colored discharges, which are more annoying than irritating. A quick week of treatment with tablets and your vaginal flora will be rebalanced.

Group B streptococcus (GBS) infections can be confused with mycosis, because they often lead to itching, and they can be a factor for vaginosis if pH increases. During pregnancy, your doctor will always look for the presence of this bacteria and, if it's detected, he or she will prescribe antibiotics during delivery to prevent the frightening GBS sepsis in newborns. Rest assured, for an adult woman, there is no danger in carrying streptococcus in the vagina.

Although they are unpleasant, the previously described vulvovaginitis infections do not endanger your health, contrary to sexually transmitted infections, which can have serious consequences.

How to Prevent Discomfort and Irritation

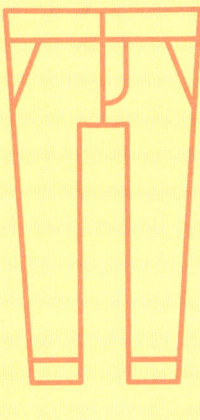

1

Avoid tight clothing (like tight jeans) and choose loose clothing. Also avoid wearing tights, which can cause microtrauma through rubbing. Moreover, persistent sweating promotes moisture and maceration (softened tissue from moisture), which can potentially cause problems.

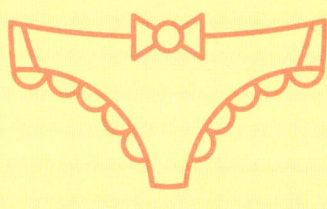

2

Wear cotton underwear and avoid synthetic materials such as nylon, which also promotes maceration.

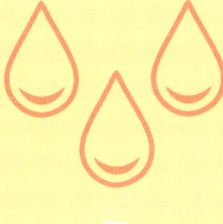

3

Avoid wearing a wet bathing suit for long periods of time. Dry yourself off quickly and put on clean, dry (cotton!) underwear as soon as possible. Moisture and maceration can encourage yeast infections.

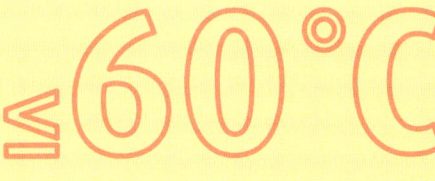

4

Wash your underwear in minimum 140°F (60°C) water and, if possible, separate them from your other clothes in the machine.

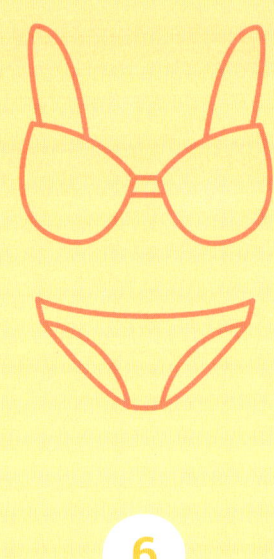

5

Do not lend your towel to anyone or borrow a towel from a friend! The same goes for your clothes, bathing suit and undergarments.

6

Change your underwear daily, even twice a day in the case of excessive sweating (for example, after playing sports, in a humid country or after a long journey, etc.).

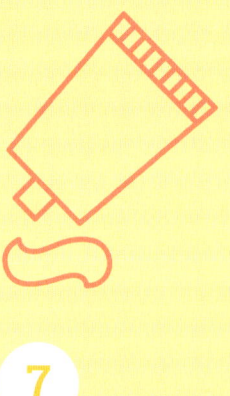

7

In case of genital discomfort (sensitivity, dryness, irritation), use a feminine hygiene wash and cream. If it doesn't improve, see your doctor.

Sexually Transmitted Infections

We'll now be discussing a more serious matter. Treatments are, of course, available, but these infections are sometimes quite insidious and fly mostly under the radar, so you don't even know they're there.

An important piece of advice: protect yourself! I've excluded AIDS and hepatitis B infections from this chapter. Although they are found in sperm and vaginal secretions, they do not produce any gynecological symptoms. In short, a simple phrase to keep in mind is "Wrap it up!" — always use a condom.

STIs can be serious. Protect yourself and get tested!

Chlamydia

Aside from two previously mentioned offenders (AIDS and hepatitis B), behold your worst enemy. Chlamydia trachomatis is a strictly sexually transmitted bacteria that often goes undetected, producing only a bit more discharge than what you likely normally experience. In men, prostatitis caused by chlamydia knows how to remain discreet. Because discharge is not itchy, foul-smelling or abnormally colored, it's likely you won't notice.

Unfortunately, if the bacteria make its way to the fallopian tubes, it's the beginning of a catastrophe. Salpingitis (infection of the fallopian tubes) can cause pelvic pain and fever or develop without symptoms. It will damage the fallopian tubes by narrowing or even blocking them, which can result in infertility or an ectopic pregnancy. Hydrosalpinx is another complication, in which the fallopian tubes become inflamed and fill with liquid.

If a diagnosis is made before this pelvic infection sets in, a simple antibiotic treatment, will prevent the situation from worsening. Your partner will also need treatment. If there's any doubt, you should get tested. The only way is by a vaginal or urethral swab; chlamydia in the cervix or in the first stream of urine indicates an infection. If that's the case, antibodies against chlamydia will appear in the blood and the serological test will be positive. Once cured, antibodies for the infection will remain positive, but it's nothing more than a marker of an old infectious episode. These antibodies do not protect against further cases, and you may be reinfected in the future. Prevention is better than cure — protect yourself!

Testing is done by a vaginal or urethral swab.

Sexually Transmitted Infections | 115

Chlamydia

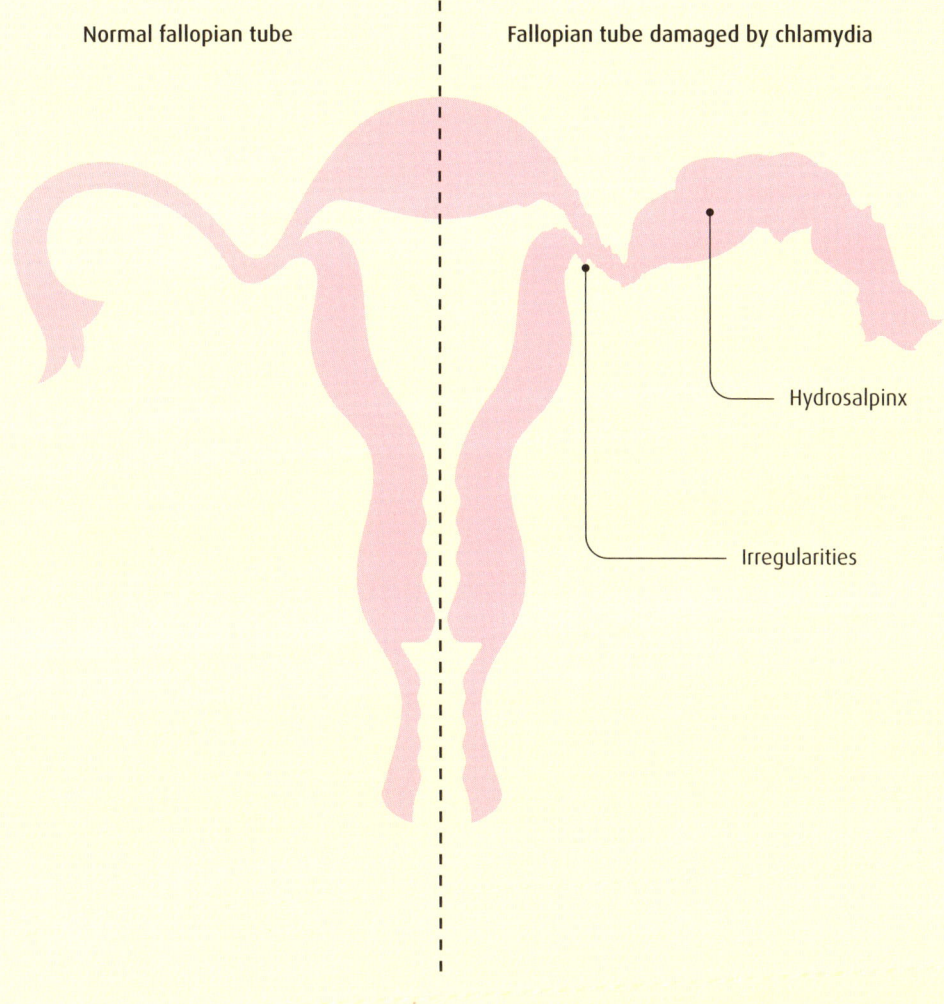

Ureaplasma and Mycoplasma Infection

Ureaplasma urealyticum and *Mycoplasma hominis* are closely related bacteria that are always tested for together. The infection caused by these bacteria is halfway between a vaginal flora imbalance and an STI. Effectively, these two bacteria can be part of vaginosis, along with their friends gardnerella and streptococcus. However, because these bacteria are also present in the prostate, they can be transmitted sexually. The infection is treated only if it causes bothersome discharge or if the number of bacteria found in a sample is greater than 10,000 per milliliter. Depending on the case, the doctor will choose to treat the partner or not.

Trichomoniasis

If one day *Trichomonas vaginalis* pays a visit to your vagina, you will never forget it. It causes green, foamy, musty-smelling discharge and a burning sensation worthy of hell fire. The vulva turns bright red and the cervix, which only a gynecologist can see, is raspberry red. Co-infections occur frequently, so trichomonas is often accompanied by other bad guys (gonococcus and chlamydia in particular). For this reason, in addition to a vaginal bacteriological swab, you will be prescribed serological tests for other STIs (HIV, hepatitis B, syphilis). There are also at-home kits that can test for candida, gardnerella and trichomonas. If there is no co-infection with a more menacing bacteria, you got off lightly. Treatment is a quick single dose for you and your partner.

Gonorrhea

Gonorrhea is caused by a bacteria called, in medical terms, *Neisseria gonorrhoeae* — otherwise known as gonococcus. Rarer than chlamydia, it is not any less harmful. It's easily recognizable by its purulent (pus-filled) discharge and causes a burning sensation during urination. It can reach your reproductive system (uterus, fallopian tubes and ovaries), with the same effects on fertility as chlamydia. Gonorrhea in men is called "the clap" in popular culture, and us doctors have learned that the sensation described by patient is like "pissing razor blades." A warning to all...

Human Papillomavirus Infection

Human papillomavirus or HPV is extremely common; every woman who has ever had sex has almost certainly been in contact with the virus. This family of viruses is made up of many serotypes in different environments: skin (warts on hands or feet), throat, anus, cervix and vulva. Thus, they are frequent guests of the human body. But let's focus on genital HPV. There are those that live out in the open on the vulva, and those that prefer to settle into the cervix and vagina.

If you have a strong immune system (lead a healthy lifestyle, get enough sleep, follow a balanced diet, do not take any long-term immunosuppressants and do not smoke) and you don't have numerous partners, HPV will likely just stick around for several months without you even noticing and then go away on its own. On the other hand, you may see condyloma (genital warts) appear on the vulva, also called cockscomb, which conjures up an image that should help you identify these very contagious venereal warts. Strictly speaking, these warts are not serious, but it is sometimes difficult to get rid of them. To do so, your best bet is your ability to fight against the infection, in other words: your immune system. When you have a poor immune system — in the case of smoking, for example — spontaneous recovery is more difficult. Your doctor can also give you a boost by prescribing creams, and he or she may recommend cryotherapy and sometimes laser treatment.

A cervical HPV infection is a different matter! The primary HPV infection goes completely unnoticed, and you will not know that you have HPV. However, if the infection lasts for many years, it can progress to cervical cancer. In fact, certain papillomaviruses are oncogenes, which means that can transform from a normal cell into a cancerous cell. Luckily, Pap smears done every three years from age 25 to 65 (consider making an appointment if you have never had one) can help detect lesions that are dysplastic well before there is a problem. The natural history of HPV suggests that in cases of mild dysplasia when the woman has a strong immune system, these anomalies can spontaneously regress, even when the infection has begun to alter cells in the cervix. Meanwhile, lesions tend to develop slowly and, even in the absence of screening (which you will now be doing if you haven't already), 10 years can separate the first signs of the virus and the appearance of cancer.

The HPV vaccine, best administered between ages 9 and 14 and before a woman's first sexual encounter, protects against 90 percent of cervical cancers, but it does not replace Pap smears. Cervical cancer is quite rare (12,984 cases in the U.S. in 2016), but it can cause abnormal bleeding in women and is easily detectable by simply getting a Pap smear regularly..

Cervical cancer screening: get a Pap smear every three years from age 25 to 65.

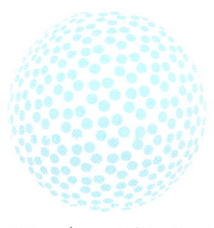
HPV under a microscope

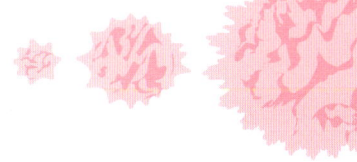
Condylomata

Genital Herpes

Of the family of herpes simplex viruses, I will be talking about oral herpes (HVS-1) and genital herpes (HVS-2). As the names imply, one mostly affects your lips up top and the other your lips down below. I say "mostly" because 30 percent of genital herpes infections are HVS-1.

I don't think I need to paint you any pictures... This infection, when it affects the vulva, is a real pain. The primary infection can be frightening: The vulva is spotted with many blisters. They are short-lived and open very quickly, resulting in painful ulcers (superficial wounds). Sometimes, the first HVS infection is not as noticeable and is just a small bunch of blisters that then become ulcers.

However, if there is a "first" infection, there will by definition be more in the future. Once someone has contracted the virus, there is no way to get rid of it. It lurks in a ganglion and as soon as it feels you are a bit under the weather, it returns with vulvar lesions, generally in the same spot as the previous attack, which heals in about a week. A treatment of valaciclovir in pill form, an antiviral medication, shortens the duration of flare-ups and increases the time between them.

Syphilis

Cases of this disease, which is caused by *Treponema pallidum* and reminds us of times gone by, are currently increasing, primarily in the male homosexual population, but no one is immune. In women, the first lesion appears as a painless ulcer, called a syphilis chancre. A large ganglion with little pain appears on the groin between four and eight days after getting infected. The chancre can occur on the vulva, vagina or cervix, as well as the mouth or throat if the infection was acquired through fellatio. It lasts for about five weeks. Beyond that, it is necessary to get a blood test for diagnosis. This is done either through routine screening or if syphilis is suspected (due to the presence of general or cutaneous signs).

Conclusion

Here we are at the end of our journey exploring the vagina!

The female genitalia may remain mysterious to some, but that no longer applies to you. Discovering your intimate anatomy, understanding it, knowing how to take care of it and enjoying it — isn't that the best way to feel like a fulfilled and complete woman?

Index

Amenorrhea **70**

Cervical mucus 26–27, 33–34, 35, 52, 73, 74

Clitoris 17, 22–**23**, 56, 60–63, 96

Conization 102–**103**

Cup, menstrual 42, 45–**46**, 71, 78

Cycle, menstrual 28–29, 32, 40–**41**, 66, 74

Cystocele 95–**96**, 100

Discharge, vaginal 26–34, 36, 53, 67, 88, 110

Dryness, vaginal 47, 48–51, 53, 70, **92**–94

Dyspareunia 85, **86**, 90

Endocrine system 43–**44**

Endometriosis 47, 86, 88–**89**

Estrogen 12, 36, 47, 48, 53, 57, 67, 68, 70, 92, 107

Fibroids 47, 104

Flora, vaginal 12, 26, 30–**31**, 32, 39, 68, 92, 106, 107–109, 116

G spot 57, 60–**62**, 63

Hormone therapy and menstruation **47**

Hysterectomy 104–**105**

Lichen sclerosus **90**

Mastodynia 47

Menopause 12, 16, 37, 48–51, 57, 78, 94, 107

Menorrhagia 47

Menstruation 26, 28–29, 32, 35, 36, **37–47**, 48, 66–67, 70–71, 73–74, 78, 88, 109

Mucus,
   Cervical 26, 33–**34**, 35, 52, 73, 74
   Ovulatory 27, 52, 67

Mycosis 90, **106**, **107**–112

Orgasm 22, 32, **56**, **57**–**61**, **63**, 84

Ovulatory mucus 27, 52, 67

Physiologic leukorrhea 26, **32**

Progestogen 47, 70

Rectocele 95–**96**, **100**

Retroverted uterus **86**–87

Surgeries 18, 85, 100–**101**, 102–105

Tampons 42–**43**, 45

Toxic Shock Syndrome 42

Transudation **32**, 36, 56

Uterus, retroverted 86–87

Vaginismus 42, **82**–**85**, 91

Vaginosis 39, 70, 73, **109**–110, 116

Vestibulitis 90, **91**

Yeast infection 90, 106, 107–112

Table of Illustrations

The Female Reproductive System (sectional view) 7

The Female Reproductive System (front view) 9

The Vagina and Perineum 11

Superficial Perineum 14

Deep Perineum 15

The Vulva 17

The Hymen Before and After the First Sexual Encounter 21

The Clitoris 23

The Walls of the Bladder, Vagina and Rectum 25

First Phase of the Cycle 28

Second Phase of the Cycle 29

Bacteria in the Vagina 31

Cervical Mucus 34

Menstrual Flow 38

The Menstrual Cycle 40–41

The Endocrine System: Our Body's Key Regulator 44

Placement of a Menstrual Cup 46

The Vagina During Childbirth 54–55

How Does an Orgasm Work? 58–59

G Spot, Where Are You? 62

Placement of a Vaginal Ring 69

Placement of an IUD in the Uterus 72

Placement of a Female Condom 77

Placement of a Diaphragm 80–81

Retroverted Uterus 87

Endometriosis 89

The Domino Effect 93

Cystocele and Rectocele 96

Prolapse 97

Prolapse Surgery 101

Conization 103

Hysterectomy 105

How to Prevent Discomfort and Irritation? 111–112

Chlamydia 115

The Author

Odile Bagot is a gynecologist and obstetrician. She has been a private practitioner for over 25 years. She holds a masters in ethics and teaches sexology at the University of Strasbourg in France. The mother of five daughters, she has been faced with all sorts of questions about the vagina. She keeps a blog (mamgyneco.wordpress.com) and Facebook page (which has 3,500 followers), and she contributes to various magazines, including Elle and Santé Magazine, and the online medical resource site Medisite. As an author and speaker, she uses an uninhibited and positive style that is also scientifically rigorous.

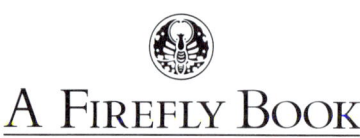

A Firefly Book

Published by Firefly Books Ltd. 2020
English translation © Firefly Books Ltd. 2020
Text © Odile Bagot 2019
Image Credit : Thinkstockphotos
© First published in French by Mango, Paris, France 2019
as *Vagin et cie, on vous dit tout* (9782317019616)

All rights reserved. No part of this publication may be reproduced, stored in a retrieval system, or transmitted in any form or by any means, electronic, mechanical, photocopying, recording or otherwise, without the prior written permission of the Publisher.

First printing

Library of Congress Control Number: 2020937809

Library and Archives Canada Cataloguing in Publication
Title: Your vagina : everything you need to know! / Odile Bagot, MD, Gynecologist.
Other titles: Vagin et cie. English
Names: Bagot, Odile, author.
Description: Includes index. | Translation of: Vagin et cie.
Identifiers: Canadiana 20200240277 | ISBN 9780228103059 (softcover)
Subjects: LCSH: Vagina—Popular works. | LCSH: Generative organs, Female—Popular works. | LCSH:
   Human reproduction—Popular works.
Classification: LCC QP259 .B3413 2020 | DDC 612.6/2—dc23

Published in Canada by
Firefly Books Ltd.
50 Staples Avenue, Unit 1
Richmond Hill, Ontario
L4B 0A7

Published in the United States by
Firefly Books (U.S.) Inc.
P.O. Box 1338, Ellicott Station
Buffalo, New York
14205

Design and Layout: Cyril Terrier
Translator: Adriana Paradiso

Printed in China

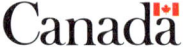 We acknowledge the financial support of the Government of Canada